**PAHC Library**

University of Plymouth

(01752) 588 588

LibraryandITenquiries@plymouth.ac.uk

# The Fast Track Program for Children at Risk

## Also Available

African American Family Life:
Ecological and Cultural Diversity
*Vonnie C. McLoyd, Nancy E. Hill, and Kenneth A. Dodge, Editors*

Aggression, Antisocial Behavior, and Violence among Girls:
A Developmental Perspective
*Martha Putallaz and Karen L. Bierman, Editors*

Cognitive-Behavioral Interventions for Emotional
and Behavioral Disorders: School-Based Practice
*Matthew J. Mayer, Richard Van Acker, John E. Lochman,
and Frank M. Gresham, Editors*

Deviant Peer Influences in Programs for Youth:
Problems and Solutions
*Kenneth A. Dodge, Thomas J. Dishion,
and Jennifer E. Lansford, Editors*

Enhancing Early Attachments:
Theory, Research, Intervention, and Policy
*Lisa J. Berlin, Yair Ziv, Lisa Amaya-Jackson,
and Mark T. Greenberg, Editors*

Helping Schoolchildren Cope with Anger, Second Edition:
A Cognitive-Behavioral Intervention
*Jim Larson and John E. Lochman*

Helping the Noncompliant Child, Second Edition:
Family-Based Treatment for Oppositional Behavior
*Robert J. McMahon and Rex L. Forehand*

Peer Rejection: Developmental Processes and Intervention Strategies
*Karen L. Bierman*

Preventing Child Maltreatment: Community Approaches
*Kenneth A. Dodge and Dorian Lambelet Coleman, Editors*

Promoting School Readiness and Early Learning:
Implications of Developmental Research for Practice
*Michel Boivin and Karen L. Bierman, Editors*

Social and Emotional Skills Training for Children:
The Fast Track Friendship Group Manual
*Karen L. Bierman, Mark T. Greenberg, John D. Coie,
Kenneth A. Dodge, John E. Lochman, and Robert J. McMahon*

Understanding Peer Influence in Children and Adolescents
*Mitchell J. Prinstein and Kenneth A. Dodge, Editors*

# The Fast Track Program for Children at Risk

## Preventing Antisocial Behavior

**Conduct Problems
Prevention Research Group**

Karen L. Bierman, John D. Coie,
Kenneth A. Dodge, Mark T. Greenberg,
John E. Lochman, Robert J. McMahon,
and Ellen E. Pinderhughes

*Foreword by Patrick H. Tolan*

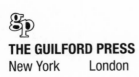

**THE GUILFORD PRESS**
New York      London

Copyright © 2020 The Guilford Press
A Division of Guilford Publications, Inc.
370 Seventh Avenue, Suite 1200, New York, NY 10001
www.guilford.com

Printed in the United States of America

This book is printed on acid-free paper.

Last digit is print number:   9   8   7   6   5   4   3   2   1

The authors have checked with sources believed to be reliable in their efforts
to provide information that is complete and generally in accord with the
standards of practice that are accepted at the time of publication. However,
in view of the possibility of human error or changes in behavioral, mental
health, or medical sciences, neither the authors, nor the editor and publisher,
nor any other party who has been involved in the preparation or publication
of this work warrants that the information contained herein is in every
respect accurate or complete, and they are not responsible for any errors or
omissions or the results obtained from the use of such information. Readers
are encouraged to confirm the information contained in this book with other
sources.

Library of Congress Cataloging-in-Publication Data is available
from the publisher.

ISBN 978-1-4625-4129-4 (hardcover)

# About the Authors

**Karen L. Bierman, PhD,** is Evan Pugh University Professor, Professor of Psychology and Human Development and Family Studies, and Director of the Child Study Center at The Pennsylvania State University. Since the 1980s, her research has focused on social-emotional development and children at risk, with an emphasis on the design and evaluation of school-based programs that promote social competence, school readiness, and positive peer relations, and that reduce aggression and related behavior problems. Currently, she directs the Research-based Developmentally Informed (REDI) classroom and home visiting programs, developed in partnership with Head Start programs in Pennsylvania. A clinical psychologist, Dr. Bierman also directs a predoctoral training program in the interdisciplinary educational sciences. Dr. Bierman has served as an educational advisor to organizations including Head Start and Sesame Workshop.

**John D. Coie, PhD,** is Professor Emeritus of Psychology and Neuroscience at Duke University. He is a past chair of the National Institute of Mental Health grant review panel on prevention research. A developmental and clinical psychologist, Dr. Coie has focused his research primarily on the development and prevention of serious antisocial behavior. He retired from Duke in 2000 but continues to be involved with the Fast Track project and has developed and comanaged a program in Santa Barbara, California, for providing non-English-speaking Hispanic children with computer-based English language and reading training. He continues to be active in programs designed to reduce violence and recidivism in the community.

**Kenneth A. Dodge, PhD,** is Pritzker Professor of Public Policy and Psychology and Neuroscience at Duke University. He is Founding and Emeritus Director of the Duke Center for Child and Family Policy. A clinical and developmental psychologist, Dr. Dodge studies early childhood development, prevention of violent behavior in the family, and public policy to improve population outcomes for communities. He is the developer of Family Connects, a population approach to improve children's outcomes in the first year of life. The author of more than 500 highly cited scientific articles, Dr. Dodge has been elected to the National Academy of Medicine and is the 2019–2021 president of the Society for Research in Child Development.

**Mark T. Greenberg, PhD,** is Emeritus Professor in the College of Health and Human Development at The Pennsylvania State University, where he is also Founding Director of the Edna Bennett Pierce Prevention Research Center. A developmental psychologist, Dr. Greenberg is the author of over 350 journal articles and book chapters on the development of well-being; learning; and the effects of prevention efforts on children and families. He is a founding board member of the Collaborative for Academic, Social, and Emotional Learning (CASEL). Dr. Greenberg is the recipient of numerous awards, including the Urie Bronfenbrenner Award for Lifetime Contribution to Developmental Psychology in the Service of Science and Society from the American Psychological Association. One of his current interests is how to help nurture awareness and compassion in our society. He is chairperson of the board of CREATE, a nonprofit devoted to improving the quality of schooling and the lives of teachers and students.

**John E. Lochman, PhD, ABPP,** is Saxon Professor Emeritus in Psychology, Interim Director of the Alabama Life Research Institute, and Director Emeritus of the Center for Prevention of Youth Behavior Problems at the University of Alabama. He is also Adjunct Professor of Psychiatry and Behavioral Sciences at Duke University Medical Center. A clinical psychologist, Dr. Lochman has authored more than 400 scientific articles, chapters, and books on the causes and consequences of highly aggressive behavior in childhood, and on the effects of intervention for this behavior. His current focus is research on dissemination, implementation, and adaptation of interventions. Dr. Lochman has served as editor-in-chief of the *Journal of Abnormal Child Psychology* and is a former president of the Society for Child and Family Policy and Practice (Division 37 of the American Psychological Association) and the American Board of Clinical Child and Adolescent Psychology. He is a recipient of the Distinguished Career Award from the Society of Clinical Child and Adolescent Psychology (Division 53 of the American Psychological Association).

**Robert J. McMahon, PhD,** is Professor of Psychology at Simon Fraser University in Burnaby, British Columbia, Canada, where he is also B.C. Leading Edge Endowment Fund Leadership Chair in Proactive Approaches to Reducing Risk for Violence among Children and Youth. To carry out the work of the chair, he directs the Institute for the Reduction of Youth Violence. He is also a senior scientist at the B.C. Children's Hospital Research Institute in Vancouver. A clinical psychologist, Dr. McMahon studies the assessment, treatment, and prevention of conduct problems and other problem behaviors in children and youth, especially in the context of the family. He is author or editor of more than 250 books, scientific articles, chapters, and reviews; a past editor-in-chief of *Prevention Science*; and a recipient of the Service to SPR Award from the Society for Prevention Research and the Trailblazer Award from the Parenting and Families Special Interest Group, Association for Behavioral and Cognitive Therapies.

**Ellen E. Pinderhughes, PhD,** is Professor in the Eliot–Pearson Department of Child Study and Human Development at Tufts University. A developmental and clinical psychologist, she studies contextual influences on and cultural processes in parenting among families facing different challenges. Dr. Pinderhughes's research interests include cultural socialization and preparation for bias among transracial adoptive parents; stigma; pathways to fatherhood and family life among gay fathers; and the role of race, ethnicity, and culture in parenting and youth outcomes. A past William T. Grant Faculty Scholar, Dr. Pinderhughes was a member of the Institute of Medicine Committee on Child Maltreatment Research, Policy, and Practice for the Next Decade: Phase II, which issued the report *New Directions in Child Abuse and Neglect Research.* She is a member of several boards focused on enhancing the lives of marginalized youth and families through research and practice.

# Foreword

In the early 1990s, there was growing public concern about increases in rates of crime, which coincided with improved documentation suggesting that violent behavior peaks during adolescence. A national review of youth delinquency and violence suggested two important patterns: (1) criminal involvement, particularly as marked by official records, was highly elevated for those growing up in the most impoverished communities, particularly urban inner-city neighborhoods, and (2) among those youth involved in crime, more than half of the total number of criminal acts were attributable to about 6% of the population (Blumstein, Cohen, Roth, & Visher, 1986). In addition, the conclusion of contemporaneous reviews about interventions to stem youth crime was that "nothing worked," although in fact there were very few quality studies illuminating what worked and what did not (Tolan & Guerra, 1994). At the same time, emerging results from longitudinal studies began to help characterize developmental typicality and pathology and to identify promising risk factors for intervention targeting. The idea was that prevention during childhood and early adolescence could target the risk and protective factors identified in longitudinal studies and alter developmental trajectories toward or away from future criminality and mental health problems (Coie et al., 1993; Kellam et al., 1991). Moreover, a substantial number of developmental and clinical scientists were eager to apply their skills and scientific methods with the goal of providing important public health benefits (Guerra, Tolan, & Hammond, 1994). A new field of prevention science was emerging to connect sophisticated analytic methods and informative empirical findings to design and evaluate preventive interventions that could address this important public health problem.

Related to this coalescence of influences, the National Institute of Mental Health (NIMH) issued a special request for proposals (RFP) requiring application of randomized controlled trial (RCT) methods to address the question of what, if anything, could be done to prevent youth violence. (The authors of the current book provide a more extensive description of the confluence of influences that set the stage for it, including identifying the visionary leadership of Doreen Koretz and others within NIMH to make prevention RCTs viable grants and to coordinate the work across groups.) The RFP included funding at a level that was exceptional at the time, making it plausible to launch studies of the scope and length needed for meaningful tests of the proposed programs. Two awards were made for large-scale prevention trials: Fast Track, which is the focus of this book, and the Metropolitan Area Child Study (MACS; Guerra, Eron, Huesmann, & Tolan, 1997), on which I collaborated with four other scientists. Each effort addressed a critical aspect of the question about the two epidemiological patterns of youth crime. Fast Track focused on those individuals who exhibited relatively high rates of aggression and other indicators of risk for conduct disorders, and the intervention was designed to start working with children and their parents at an early age. MACS focused on inner-city and urban poor communities where overall rates were elevated, with a school-based universal intervention as its core, as well as group and family interventions for students with elevated aggression levels. While quite different in many key ways, these projects overlapped in their efforts to bring developmental science into complex interventions tested through longitudinal evaluation of RCTs. One requirement of the funding was a willingness to work collaboratively across projects, to share ideas and strategies for full implementation as well as to consider measurement consistency. As a result, I had the opportunity to become acquainted with the people conducting Fast Track, scholars for whom I had a great deal of admiration, and with whom I began a decades-long collegial relationship including ongoing familiarity with this very important project.

Fast Track has become one of the most influential research studies in prevention in the past three decades. There is extensive evidence of the importance of Fast Track for improving our ability to address conduct disorder, which is one of the most intractable and most prevalent of mental health problems in children; for linking the development approach of prevention of this problem to broad and substantial benefits in preventing violent crime, mental illness, and substance use; and in serving as a groundbreaking and model effort in conducting prevention science. This exceptionally talented and dedicated group of scientists took on one of the most challenging scientific projects imaginable from both practical and logistical angles. They were able to implement a complementary and carefully developed set of intervention components. They accomplished this through excellent fidelity, clear theoretical formulations, intimate knowledge of the real-world challenges, and concern for the communities in which the project was conducted. The sustained level of effort and the resulting publications and policy-relevant solutions related to child and youth mental health and behavior issues emanating from Fast Track is, to date, unparalleled in the field of prevention. This culminating volume provides detailed and forthcoming results and discussions addressing the myriad important questions that are part of understanding conduct disorder, what can be done to prevent it and further problems related to it later in life, how to best accomplish needed implementation, and how to locate all these findings and implications within the larger science of prevention and public health interest in reducing mental illness and criminal behavior rates. In addition, for those pursuing developmental science, it is a model of how to apply our science to test causally sophisticated formulations.

Starting with an overview and careful articulation of the circumstances leading to the project and the theory driving the integration of multiple intervention components, the book then provides an in-depth look into a set of logically successive topics that help answer several wide-ranging questions:

Did it work?
How did it work?
For whom did it work?
How are effects different at different life stages?
What is the impact on the ultimate outcome of adult crime and mental health?
What did not go as hoped/planned?
And, finally, what might this mean for other scientists, practitioners, and policy makers?

At each juncture, with each topic, the volume helps the reader understand why the science was conducted the way it was, what the basic findings were (expected and unexpected), and what the nuances within those basic patterns were. It also provides guidance as to the implications for prevention science, for developmental understanding, and for addressing the lives of these high-risk children and their families.

Throughout this extensive report of data-based results are integrated case studies to highlight and focus on the human lives and the personal impact represented in those data. Furthermore, the authors elaborate upon what the findings might mean for similar efforts or for next-stage studies. These nuanced and technical details are made accessible to readers of diverse backgrounds and those with varying familiarity with the project as well as the topics at hand. The material can be read from the perspective of a scientist, a practitioner, or a policy-interested professional. The volume accomplishes what is rarely achieved: It provides a full investigation of effects of a prevention effort with translation to practical implications and thoughtful linking to what follows.

The volume provides much that is notable and worth exploring in detail. I highlight just a few of the rich examples to illustrate the depth and breadth of the findings. First, the final outcomes reporting is fundamentally important for our society and worthy of scaling up: 31% reduction in rates of violence, 35% reduction in drug abuse, lower rates of internalizing problems (anxiety and depression), and lower rates of externalizing problems (conduct disorder, antisocial personality). A concern often raised as a criticism of the Fast Track effort was that it was so extensive and costly it would not be replicable in practice nor justifiable. A basic principle guiding the project was the social and economic worth regarding this investment of concentrated resources targeting multiple developmental domains over most of childhood and adolescence. The results justify this concentration of effort and the related service structure and investment requirements. It is important to keep in mind that this program targeted the subgroup of children most likely to engage in serious delinquency, fail at school, and populate our jails. As the cost–benefit analyses show, if implemented in a focused and sustained manner, this intervention results in substantial savings to our society by preventing the need for more intensive and costly criminal justice, educational, and mental health services and in avoiding costs to others that otherwise would result. As noted in this book, however, the political will to focus resources in this manner is a critical missing ingredient for future dissemination of the Fast Track model. Notably, variants of this model, which have found ways to reduce the cost of the intervention, are being launched and evaluated to provide a concession to practicality. However, as tested and reported about here, we have a prevention approach proven to effect substantially important outcomes for children at high risk for conduct disorder. We know it will pay dividends for them, their families, and those who live in their communities.

Second, while there are meaningful variations among subgroups in terms of the extent and nature of the outcomes that showed benefits, the prevailing pattern is consistency of effects. Similarly, the benefits of the original Fast Track program varied at different times during development, but patterns of effects showed general consistency across gender, residence location, ethnicity, and socioeconomic status. As the authors carefully note, this is not to suggest that there are not important variations within these overall patterns, nor that the life course of children can be understood apart from political and social forces and inequities. The report integrates attention to political and social standing differences and micro and macro contextual influences in interpreting results and in suggesting limitations of what can be learned from this work. For example, the results suggest that the impact on adolescent substance use is limited to white adolescents, not showing significance at that point in development for black youth. However, this is in accord with epidemiological findings that during adolescence, substance use differs among these two populations. The racial/ethnic difference in effects is important but may reflect how base rates can affect potential preventive benefits. A different understanding emerges about cognitive targets during elementary school. Here, the benefits are not extended to those from more disadvantaged socioeconomic levels. As is too often the case, promoting beneficial boosts in the development of resilience skills may be most difficult in youth facing the most challenging environments. These patterns and the discussion herein are not meant to indicate that one size fits all or that important markers of differences in social and political standing and opportunity are not relevant to conduct disorder. However, among the most at risk within a given population, these strategies seem valuable and the components assembled comprise a useful prevention effort for a broad constituency—one that is context informed and adjusted to fit the social ecology of those engaged.

Third, this study supports the notion that development can be viewed as a cascade of transactions between the individual proclivities at a given point in time and accumulating experiences and contexts. These interactions lead to variations in unfolding probabilities of greater positivity or negativity going forward. In essence, the extent to which we nurture and support youth early in development sets a course that, while not predetermined, makes future directions substantially more or less likely. At the same time, this study also demonstrates how dynamic and heterogeneous developmental cascades can occur based on shifts in life-course circumstances and opportunities, even for those entering school with some of the most pessimistic expectations. An unexpected finding is the heterogeneity in trajectories of those identified as high risk, apart from intervention influence. The provision of empirical information and extensive exploration of multiple aspects of key influences and settings over critical years of development provide a rich and compelling argument for the value of early intervention and for optimism about youth, even those most at risk. Further credence is lent by the findings that in addition to reducing rates of crime and mental illness, the Fast Track prevention efforts produced higher rates of positive functioning indicators such as well-being, happiness, civic engagement, and participation in voting.

Fourth, the work that went into conducting this study is a model for prevention scientists (including public health and clinical intervention scientists) in how to conduct research and bring it to fruition. Admittedly, this was a very accomplished group prior to forming the collaboration that brought together a heretofore unparalleled breadth of skills. They were able to secure unprecedented levels of funding and sustain the study over a length of time few other projects have. Having witnessed this research firsthand, I can say that what they have produced is fundamentally about the care and critical review they applied to each step, the willingness to listen to others' advice and incorporate new knowledge and methods thoughtfully, and the ability to show the scientific and public health value of the work at each stage.

While leading the field in many ways, this group also engaged with others to enable them to benefit from their skills and knowledge, spurring the field on in a broader way. At the outset of this work, there was emerging recognition that conducting RCTs to track preventive effects was a new type of scientific work. What became evident immediately was that it would require ongoing learning, formulating specific challenges not evident in adjacent fields or from prior limited efforts. It also required engaging others, particularly methodologists, to help build analytic capabilities along with theory advancements and increasingly complex data sets. This is one of several efforts that were part of that exciting period of rapid development for prevention efforts. Karen Bierman, John Coie, Kenneth Dodge, Mark Greenberg, John Lochman, Robert McMahon, and Ellen Pinderhughes each individually contributed to that transformative effort, but through Fast Track they were trailblazers in their ability to collaborate as a team, producing contributions greater than the sum of the individual efforts. For example, they were the first to use the corporate name, Conduct Problems Prevention Research Group, which put the collaboration at the center of citations, not the individuals. That was the direct inspiration for our Metropolitan Area Child Study and Multisite Violence Prevention Project corporate authorships.

Not surprisingly, this volume ends by noting the limitations of the project and offering suggestions for next steps in prevention science. It also offers advice for decreasing the prevalence of violence and improving outcomes for those showing conduct problems early in life. These limitations, followed by larger implications, should help readers properly use this volume, whether seeking direction for research, trying to determine what prevention effort to implement in one's community, or trying to encourage policies that could be informed by this work. Two important lessons that have come to rest with me over my career, which

I try to instill in my students, are represented in the conclusions. First, scientific study, and especially RCTs, are blunt instruments that can, by focusing on and simplifying what is being tested, provide insight and confidence about details that are almost impossible to gain otherwise. Yet, this simplification is necessary. The complex ecology of behavior and the way development is altered must be treated more simply than it usually is, and some aspects have to be overlooked or treated as secondary. As has been said about democracy being the worst form of government except all the rest, RCTs of this quality and scale are a limited way to soundly advance knowledge for improving mental health, but are better than all the other alternatives. Second, as veterans of developmental tracking studies know from painful experience, often longitudinal research is learning what you should have measured. By extension, I would say RCTs are often about learning what you should (or should not) have emphasized in your prevention efforts. While the Fast Track study has not escaped these sobering aspects of such work entirely, it certainly has managed to minimize them and to fulfill its promise with enviable foresight and capability. In addition to what was learned about what should or should not have been done, this project's accomplishments set a firm base for subsequent efforts.

This volume presents an opportunity to learn about prevention science, prevention as public good, and the ways our society can fundamentally and substantially alter our nonproductive punitive focus on children who come to our classrooms with behavior problems, seemingly destined for troubled and troubling lives. There are lessons for all here in this compelling presentation. I look forward to seeing how its availability and use spurs progress in science, practice, and policy— one more fundamental and groundbreaking contribution from the Fast Track program.

PATRICK H. TOLAN, PHD
*University of Virginia*

## REFERENCES

Blumstein, A., Cohen, J., Roth, J. A., & Visher, C. A. (Eds.). (1986). *Criminal careers and "career criminals."* Washington, DC: National Academy Press.

Coie, J. D., Watt, N. F., West, S. G., Hawkins, J. D., Asarnow, J. R., Markman, H. J., . . . Long, B. (1993). The science of prevention: A conceptual framework and some directions for a national research program. *American Psychologist, 48*(10), 1013–1022.

Guerra, N. G., Eron, L. D., Huesmann, L. R., & Tolan, P. H. (1997). A cognitive-ecological approach to the prevention and mitigation of violence and aggression in inner-city youth. In D. P. Fry & K. Björkqvist (Eds.), *Cultural variation in conflict resolution: Alternatives to violence* (pp. 199–213). Hillsdale, NJ: Erlbaum.

Guerra, N. G., Tolan, P. H., & Hammond, W. R. (1994). Prevention and treatment of adolescent violence. In L. D. Eron, J. H. Gentry, & P. Schlegel (Eds.), *Reason to hope: A psychosocial perspective on violence and youth* (pp. 383–403). Washington, DC: American Psychological Association.

Kellam, S., Werthamer-Larsson, L., Dolan, J. L., Brown, H., Mayer, L., Rebok, G., . . . Wheeler, L. (1991). Developmental epidemiologically based preventive trials: Baseline modeling of early target behaviors and depressive symptoms. *American Journal of Community Psychology, 19,* 563–584.

Tolan, P. H., & Guerra, N. (1994). *What works in reducing adolescent violence: An empirical review of the field.* Boulder: Center for the Study and Prevention of Violence, Institute for Behavioral Sciences, University of Colorado, Boulder.

# Preface

The seven of us who conducted the Fast Track prevention trial recognize the enormous privilege that has been ours—one that may not be offered again soon, if ever. To be able to test the hypothesis that a multifaceted early intervention can prevent adolescent and young adult crime and violence has been a remarkable opportunity for us, given the funding to include large numbers of at-risk youth from varying geographic locales across a time span from school entry through adolescence into the adult years. We are grateful to the many people and agencies that made it possible, not all of whom could possibly be mentioned in this Preface.

Several factors converged to create the unique circumstances supporting this undertaking. One of these was the upsurge of crime, particularly violent crime, in the mid to late 1980s that motivated public interest in and commitment to prevention programming. A second factor was the coming to fruition of several important longitudinal studies of child behavior problems that illuminated early risk factors and identified key developmental processes associated with future crime and violence. Third, prevention programs were demonstrating the capacity to produce short-term improvements in specific parent, child, or school factors linked longitudinally with future crime and violence. Together, these studies highlighted critical risk factors to target in prevention programming, demonstrated the malleability of these risk factors and the feasibility of various prevention approaches, and laid the groundwork for a more comprehensive and intensive approach to prevention that might have long-term benefits for high-risk children and youth. These three factors formed the background for Fast Track.

In the late 1980s, program officers at the National Institute of Mental Health (NIMH) began to host conferences to discuss prevention programming for youth exhibiting antisocial behavior. One of them, Doreen Koretz, had a singular role in the realization of the Fast Track project. Initially she convened investigators who had conducted some of the longitudinal and prevention studies just mentioned. In one such instance, she assembled a small group to discuss future directions that NIMH and related agencies might take to pull together what was then known about causes of and remedies for antisocial behavior into an integrated longer-term prevention trial. More than anyone else, Doreen should be given credit for nurturing the efforts that supported the design and eventual implementation of Fast Track. Others, such as John Reid and Debra Pepler, who had themselves made important contributions to the science of preventing antisocial behavior, were particularly supportive of this effort. Chapter 1 provides an expanded account of this history, and Chapter 2 provides more detail regarding the individuals whose research and ideas framed the theory underlying Fast Track and the prevention strategies that we employed.

The communities in which Fast Track was carried out were selected on the basis of their proximity to investigators who had experience in prevention programming for aggressive youth and because they provided geographic and population diversity for the large-scale evaluation. Schools were taken as the starting point for finding high-risk youth in each of the four geographic areas. Those serving populations of generally low-income and high-crime prevalence were asked to participate, with the understanding that some would be randomly selected for the prevention trial and others for the control group sample. It was not always easy to get administrators to make this commitment, and one of the ongoing issues for the project was to keep school system collaboration ongoing despite changes in administration. Thus, we are extremely appreciative of and grateful for the administrative support that Fast Track received and the continuous participation of schools at each of the four sites.

Fast Track included multicomponent, cross-context (home–school) prevention activities carried out over a 10-year period. One of the challenges we struggled with in this design involved annual decisions regarding how best to meet what we perceived as the child, family, and school needs at each developmental level, on the one hand, and the realistic limits of resources to support prevention programming. In an ideal prevention process, protective factors are successfully strengthened and risk factors are successfully reduced at an early stage, reducing future child and family need for intervention support. In reality, many of the children and families who participated in Fast Track lived in extremely challenging circumstances in which unpredictable twists of fate led to unstable upswings or significant downturns in child and family functioning. Our prevention plan included gradual reductions in the frequency of intervention sessions over time. For some parents, this prevention program pacing was adequate to meet their needs. Yet, for many others, issues such as handling discipline problems (which were a primary focus of the first 2 years) continued to be a challenge for many subsequent years, sparking requests to revisit the early prevention topics in later years. In the chapters of this book, we provide an overview of the prevention programming that Fast Track utilized across its 10-year span, along with the individualized tailoring that was developed to address the range of family needs. Several case studies are followed throughout the book to provide an illustration of the varying patterns of child and family response to the program.

Something we did not fully anticipate at the start of Fast Track was the way in which apparent progress with reducing children's behavior problems did not always manifest itself immediately, and sometimes not for several years. The early grade school years reflected many of the positive changes we hoped for. Middle school was, in contrast, much more disappointing in terms of behavioral improvements. For one thing, we had less contact with parents and very little contact with teachers because individual teachers had no sustained contact with students.

Things began to come into better accordance with our original goals during the high school and succeeding years, after formal Fast Track programming had ended. The fact that we were able to attain the magnitude of reductions in disruptive and criminal behavior that we did, as well as positive mental health outcomes emerging in the early adult years of program participants, proved the viability of our developmental premises and our program. These results were a source of both relief and celebration for the seven of us and our staffs, and are described in chapters summarizing the findings at each core developmental phase (elementary school, middle school, high school, and early adulthood).

In the final chapters of the book, we discuss more specifically the challenges to be faced in designing effective prevention programming of this kind in the future, and our thoughts about how these challenges might be handled. Our hope, and the purpose of this volume, is that the Fast Track project will serve as an impetus for the advancement of science on the development and prevention of violence and crime and for more widespread and innovative community efforts to reduce these problems. After paying for preparation expenses, additional royalties from this book are being donated to the Society for Prevention Research to support ongoing developments in prevention science.

# Acknowledgments

There are many people who must be acknowledged for their role in making Fast Track a success. Space does not permit mentioning everyone, but the following individuals participated for an extended time in major roles at one or more of the four sites.

At the Durham site, Donna Marie Winn was the Clinical Supervisor. Christina Christopoulos, Jeff Quinn, and Melissa Martin were Research Coordinators. Leslie Fair Grey, Marchell Gunter, Gann Herman, Jackie Parrish, Bernadette Simpson-Berry, and Alfreida Stevens were Family Coordinators. Moss Cohen, Jean Geratz, Mara Gleason, Deborah Jones, Shelley Legall Brickey, and Anthony Miller were Educational Coordinators. Willie Burt, Ivan Evans, Jonathan Gattis, Clarine Hyman, Malik Lee, and Trevor Peterson were Youth Coordinators. Dustin Albert, Max Crowley, Reid Fontaine, Mary Gifford-Smith, Tom Hannon, Julie Kaplow, Patrick Malone, Ann Maumary-Gremaud, Shari Miller, Melba Nicholson, David Rabiner, Lucy Sorensen, and Elizabeth Stearns were Data Analysts. Administrative and Senior Research Staff were Bea Chestnut, Tammie Harbison, Donna Hubert, Ocie Ingram, Denice Johnson, Annie Jones, Rosalie Parrish, Phyllis Peacock, Jolyn Peck, Theresa Renuart, Karen Novy, and Barbara Pollock.

At the Nashville site, Alison Fuller was an Educational Coordinator and Youth Coordinator before becoming the site Principal Investigator. Sheila Peters was a Clinical Supervisor. Janice Brown, Joan Deer, and Erin Tomarken were Research Coordinators. Marilyn Bell, Benita Collins, Shirley Davis Brooks, Mary Jo Heimbigner, Beverly Mahan, Shirley Nix Davis, Janet Shands, and Beverly Taylor were Family Coordinators and/or Youth Coordinators. Deidra Adamczyk, Maggie Amditis, Kenettha Ellis, Laurie Erickson, Todd Jackson, Beverly Jacobs, Dorothy

Morelli, Purvis Preshá, Wayne Tiller, Troy Wade, and Beth Williams were Educational Coordinators and/or Youth Coordinators. Jilah Khalil and Janice Shavers were Research Staff. Data Analysts included Jennifer Harnish, Laura Griner Hill, Sean Hurley, Damon Jones, Chase Lesane-Brown, Stephanie Milan, Robert Nix, Joan Orrell-Valente, David Schwartz, Judith Scott, Joseph Wehby, and Arnaldo Zelli. Becky Bembry and Lynn Clayton Jones were Administrative Staff.

At the Pennsylvania site, Jessianne McCarthy, Richard Plut, and Gloria Rhule were Clinical Supervisors. Janet Welsh supervised the mentor program. Carole Bruschi and Sandra Stewart were Research Supervisors. Sheila Barlock, Kathleen Fenchak, Madeline Gill, Jean Lundy, Holly Signarello, Susan Slaybaugh, and Julie Rauli were Family Coordinators and, in some cases, also Youth Coordinators. Elaine Berrena, Kathy Bryon, Rosemary Demer, Dorothy Piekielek, Edwina Pollock, Susan Ruth, Sandra Stewart, Dixie Svec, and Kerry Weissman were Educational Coordinators and, in some cases, also Youth Coordinators. Michael Bercaw, Robert Franz, Gregory Hall, Lisa Knudson, James Koller, Andrew Mitchell, Thomas Signarello, and John Waldron were Mentors and, in some cases, also Youth Coordinators. Floyd Hummel and Anne Clarke were Data Managers. Grace Yan Fang, Brenda Heinrichs, Damon Jones, Chi-Ming Kam, Mary Klute, Frank Lawrence, and Robert Nix were Data Analysts. Anne Keckler, Pamela Luttman, Tracy Spalvins, and Cinda Rockey were Administrative Staff.

At the Seattle site, Nancy Slough was the Project Coordinator and a Clinical Supervisor. Sandra Lahn was the Research Coordinator. Kathi Morton, Christa Turksma, and Markos Weiss were Clinical Supervisors. Susan Brower, Carolyn Davis, Walterine French, Mary Kratz, Monica Rose, Sharon Sobers-Outlaw, and Ada Thomas were Family Coordinators. Shirley Mae Anderson, Tamara Anderson, Doug Cheney, Cassie Compton, Tina Fleming, Wendy Hamlin, Janelle Hargesheimer, Micheal Kane, Harris Levinson, Donna Manion, Suze Millman, Carrie Richard, Kerri Schloredt, and Beth Vorhaus were Educational Coordinators. Tim Chambers, Walterine French, Janelle Hargesheimer, Mary Kratz, Donna Manion, Carrie Richard, and Victor Wood were Youth Coordinators. Christina Gould, Laura Payne, and Pervis Willis were Mentor/Vocational Coordinators. Suzanne Doyle, Natalie Goulter, Andrew Hummel, Erin Ingoldsby, Karen Jones, Hyoshin Kim, Liliana Lengua, Craig Mason, Carolyn McCarty, Katie Witkiewitz, and Johnny Wu were Data Analysts. Administrative Staff were Yuri Clancy, Jana Hirata, and Shan McCullough.

The Data Center was originally located in Nashville and later moved to Durham. The Data Center was led by Pamela Ahrens, Jennifer Godwin, Robert Laird, Clara Muschkin, and Ernest Valente. The staff included Jacqueline Britt, Anne Corrigan, Sharon Eatmon, Beth Gifford,

Ben Goodman, Laura Griner Hill, Ali Gusberg, Jamie Hanson, Anne-Marie Iselin, Sharon Kersteter, Patrick Malone, Larry Perry, Cindy Rains, Gary Rains, Mariscia Reid, Manan Roy, Jose Sandoval, David Schwartz, Amanda Sherrard, Zvi Strassberg, Joy Stutts, and Donald Woodley.

There were several people who were important collaborators on the project at different times with respect to the intervention and to research design and analysis. Carolyn Webster-Stratton graciously allowed us to use selected video vignettes from her Incredible Years parenting program in the Parent Groups. Members of the Social Development Research Group (SDRG) at the University of Washington (especially Kevin Haggerty, Richard Catalano, David Hawkins, and Kathy Burgoyne) allowed us to adapt content from several of their family-based interventions for use in the Parent Groups. Barbara Wasik provided consultation on the home-visiting component and we used her manual (Wasik, Bryant, & Lyons, 1990) in training the Family Coordinators. Daphna Oyserman allowed us to adapt her School to Jobs program for use during the adolescent phase of the intervention. With respect to research design and analysis, Michael Foster helped us understand the complexities of cost–benefit analyses, and Patrick Curran assisted with the conceptualization of longitudinal analyses. Linda Collins and Susan Murphy provided valuable statistical advice to us as the project matured, particularly with regard to the analysis of the adaptive elements of the program. Danielle Dick led efforts to collect DNA and conduct genetic analyses. A number of other consultants deserve our thanks for the advice they provided in areas of intervention (Kenneth Hardy, Sonja Schoenwald, Margaret Beale Spencer, and Howard Stevenson) and analyses (Mark Appelbaum, Steven Barnett, Mark Cohen, Helen Ladd, and Robert Plotnick).

We are grateful for the close collaboration of the Durham Public Schools, the Metropolitan Nashville Public Schools, the Bellefonte Area Schools, the Tyrone Area Schools, the Mifflin County Schools, the Highline Public Schools, and the Seattle Public Schools. We want to thank the families in our project for their participation and the young people who have agreed to remain participants in the numerous follow-up projects and data collections since they came of legal age.

This work would not have occurred without the support of U.S. federal agencies. Fast Track was supported by National Institute of Mental Health (NIMH) Grants R18MH48043, R18MH50951, R18MH50952, R18MH50953, R01MH062988, K05MH00797, and K05MH01027; National Institute on Drug Abuse (NIDA) Grants R01DA016903, K05DA15226, RC1DA028248, and P30DA023026; and Department of Education Grant S184U30002. The Center for Substance Abuse Prevention also provided support through a memorandum of agreement with the NIMH.

# Contents

# The Fast Track Program for Children at Risk

# Chapter 1

# Setting the Context
# for Youth Violence Prevention

It was 1989. The media was starting to report stories of teenagers who committed gruesome murders. School shootings were on the rise. On September 26, 1988, at a school in Greenwood, South Carolina, a teenage boy shot and killed an 8-year-old girl and wounded eight other children with a 9-round .22 caliber pistol. He then shot a teacher who tried to stop him and entered a third-grade classroom, wounding six more students before he was restrained. On December 16, 1988, in Virginia Beach, Virginia, a 15-year-old boy opened fire at school, wounding a teacher who fell to the ground. He then stood over her and killed her point blank. On January 17, 1989, in Stockton, California, when Patrick Edward Purdy's mother refused to give him money for drugs, he went to Cleveland School and shot over 100 rounds into the schoolyard, killing 5 students and wounding 30 more before taking his own life. On July 18, 1990, the *New York Times* carried a front-page headline, "Number of Killings Soars in Big Cities Across U.S." Two weeks later, the U.S. Senate Judiciary Committee released a report stating that the number of murders in the United States would reach an all-time high that year.

It was in this context that the National Institute of Mental Health (NIMH) realized that it needed to take quick and decisive action to address the growing concerns about rising levels of youth violence in the United States. As the lead U.S. federal agency for research on mental disorders, NIMH focused on preventing conduct disorder (CD)—the mental illness associated with youth aggression and violence. It convened meetings of experts and called for proposals to create new, innovative approaches to the prevention of CD. A group of psychologists from four different universities, calling themselves the Conduct Problems Prevention Research Group (CPPRG), responded to the call with a proposal to create a new school- and family-based intervention program, called Fast Track. The goal was to implement Fast Track in four different U.S. communities and to evaluate its impact on young children with the most rigorous scientific method available, a randomized controlled trial. That proposal was approved, beginning a 29-year project illustrating the ways in which university-based developmental science can be used to address a complex, real-world problem. This book tells that story.

## RISE IN YOUTH CRIME IN THE 1980s

Hard data verified the fact that crime in America was indeed rising in the 1980s, especially youth crime, and in particular, violent youth crime. The overall violent crime rate in the United States increased by 470% between 1960 and 1991, the year that the Fast Track randomized trial began. In addition, more and more of these crimes were being perpetrated by teenagers under the age of 18. In the period between 1980 and 1993, the rate of victim-reported violent crimes by youth increased by 49%. During the same period, the arrest rate for violent crime by children ages 10–17 increased by 68%, as shown in Figure 1.1.

Multiple factors contributed to this rise in youth crime. Albert Blumstein (1995) and other notable criminologists argued that the rise in crime was attributable to a growing crack cocaine drug trade in which urban teenagers were being recruited as drug-runners and participants. This explanation was consistent with the data, which showed the most dramatic rises in violent crime occurring among teenagers. Although murder rates by adults over the age of 24 did not change over this time, there were dramatic increases in murders committed by teenagers ages 15–18. In fact, during the short period between 1985 and 1992, the murder arrest rate among teenagers increased by over 200%, while the murder arrest rate for adults over age 30 actually declined. There was indeed a frightening problem developing with teenage violence.

At this same time, there was a sharp increase in guns being brought onto the campuses of public schools. According to a survey at that time by the Harvard School of Public Health, 15% of high school students reported that they had carried a handgun on their person in the past 30 days, and 4% reported that they had taken a handgun to school in the past year. The public school was becoming a more dangerous place.

Fueled by these statistics and sensationalized media reports, the Centers for Disease Control and Prevention (CDC) listed "Violence and Abusive Behavior" as one of 22 public health priority areas in its 1990 report of targets for Healthy People 2000 (Public Health Service,

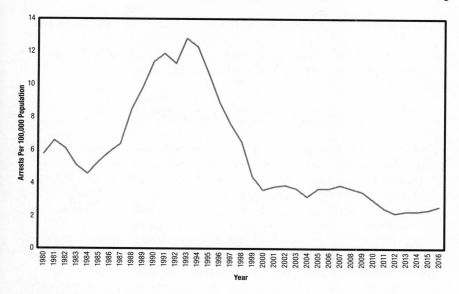

**FIGURE 1.1.** Violent crime offenses: Arrests of persons ages 10–17 per 100,000 persons ages 10–17 in the resident population. The Violent Crime Index includes the offenses of murder and nonnegligent manslaughter, rape, robbery, and aggravated assault. From OJJDP Statistical Briefing Book (n.d.). Data source: Arrest estimates developed by the Bureau of Justice Statistics and disseminated through its online "Arrest Data Analysis Tool."

1990). In 1992, a landmark issue of the prestigious scientific publication *Journal of the American Medical Association* was devoted to violent behavior, which it declared to be "a major public health problem" (Marwick, 1992, p. 2993). A year later, the CDC established the Division of Violence Prevention, one of three divisions within the newly created National Center for Injury Prevention and Control, and it publicly called the problem of violence an "epidemic" in its report, "The Prevention of Youth Violence: A Framework for Community Action." Attention was focusing on the subset of chronically aggressive teenagers.

Scholars at that time began to focus on the fact that a relatively small number of youth accounted for a large proportion of the teen crimes being committed. For example, in a long-term study of children born in Philadelphia in 1945, a select group (7%) was responsible for over half of the adolescent crimes committed (Tracy, Wolfgang, & Figlio, 1990). The adolescents most likely to commit multiple crimes were those who, as children, displayed frequent behavior problems. In fact, in a long-term study of adolescent delinquency, Robins (1978) found that approximately half of children of early school age (ages 6 or 7) who displayed frequent problem behaviors went on to engage in adolescent crime. These two findings led researchers to conclude that efforts to prevent serious adolescent crime might need to start in early elementary school and focus on children displaying early signs of aggressive behaviors.

## THE COST OF A CHRONIC CRIMINAL

In addition to the physical danger violent adolescents represented to others, there was mounting evidence that youth who committed violent crimes cost society a great deal of money. Aside from the costs for medical and emotional treatment needed by victims and their families, the violent teenagers themselves incurred costs for adjudication, incarceration, and treatment. In addition, these youth were often costly to society in other ways, including unemployment or underemployment (income taxes that they would not pay) and need for welfare or other forms of public assistance. Mark Cohen, an economist at Vanderbilt University, first reported in 1988 that the actual cost of crime was larger than anyone had assumed. He has since estimated the lifetime total cost to society of the average chronic criminal to be more than $4.2 million (Cohen & Piquero, 2009).

In the late 1980s, public interest in understanding the cost–benefit ratios for social programs was emerging. The high cost of chronic criminals set a high bar for the amount of money that might be spent on prevention efforts and still yield a positive financial return on investments, if the expenses associated with chronic patterns of violent crime were averted or reduced. Emerging longitudinal research was suggesting that the very large lifetime costs of chronic violent crime were mostly the result of the actions of children who started their antisocial behavior early in life and continued it throughout most of their lives. By the late 1980s it was also clear that it was possible to identify a pattern of early childhood misconduct that predicted with about 50% accuracy those children who would commit a disproportionate amount of juvenile violence and other crimes and continue to do so well into adulthood at an enormous cost to society. By the late 1980s all of these facts were known to the federal agencies concerned with youth violence.

## THE CALL FOR A SOLUTION

The CDC report called for innovation in prevention and treatment that would require cooperation and integration across public health, health care, mental health, criminal justice, social service, education, and other relevant sectors. In 1990, NIMH focused a spotlight on the underlying mental health problems associated with CD, characterized by an early-starting pattern of persistent aggression, and allocated funds for research examining the causes and for testing prevention programs aimed at reducing chronically aggressive and antisocial behavior by children.

The NIMH perspective was that children who were at high risk for displaying serious CD might be identified early, before their patterns of behavior became intractable. If effective preventive intervention plans could be developed to address the causes of their emergent pattern of antisocial behavior, future aggression and criminal activity might be averted or substantially reduced. The Fast Track prevention program was based on this model, in the hope that early preventive efforts with the child, the family, and the school could alter the developmental pathway toward serious CD.

While rare, this was not the first time that large-scale efforts to prevent serious adolescent crime and violence had been attempted. In 1935, little was known about the developmental features of aggression and violence, but Richard Cabot, a Boston physician, combined the legal clout of the Boston courts with the clinical wisdom of the Judge Baker Guidance Center to begin the Cambridge–Somerville Youth Study. The study became the largest attempt to date to prevent delinquency in children. Cabot was skeptical about the ability of the human services profession, especially social work, to undo damage resulting from poverty and the stress of the Great Depression, work that he likened to "attacking a granite fortress with a pea shooter" (1931, p. 8). In contrast, he had hope that the provision of preventive intervention might shape the development of vulnerable children in more positive directions.

Drawing on ongoing research on delinquency by William Healy and Augusta Bronner (1948) and the longitudinal studies of Sheldon and Eleanor Glueck (1930), the Cambridge–Somerville Youth Study program was a community-based effort to prevent delinquency. In all, 506 boys ages 5–13 in the local community signed up for the program. Cabot began a randomized controlled trial in 1939, which enrolled children for 5 years. The children assigned to the intervention received family counseling twice a month, individual tutoring, medical and psychological therapy, and a group-based summer camp program, and they were connected with a number of social service agencies. The control group received only an initial assessment.

During the first several years, the intervention team was pleased with its program. It seemed that children had benefited. But the optimism waned as the children grew older. In 1978, Joan McCord followed up with the boys who had participated in the Cambridge–Somerville Youth

Study. The findings were startling. On the measures collected, including criminal record, alcoholism, mental illness, age at death, health problems, and job status, not only was there no evidence of improvement in the intervention group, but that group was significantly worse off than the control group on several indicators. The program had no positive effect on juvenile and adult arrest rates measured by official or unofficial records. There were no differences between the two groups in the number of serious crimes committed, the age at which a first crime was committed, or the age of desistance from crime. A larger proportion of criminals from the treatment group went on to commit additional crimes than their counterparts in the control group. Boys who had been assigned to the intervention group were more likely than controls to have received serious psychiatric diagnoses, such as schizophrenia. Boys assigned to the intervention group were more likely to die at younger ages than boys in the control group. This news deflated the clinical community and became ammunition for those skeptics who favored the early detection, rounding up, and incarceration of delinquent children.

A generation passed and a second attempt, called the St. Louis Experiment, was led by Ronald Feldman, a social work professor at Washington University (Feldman, Caplinger, & Wodarski, 1983). In 1970, he and his colleagues developed a group-based therapeutic intervention to prevent antisocial behavior in boys. He randomly assigned 263 early adolescent high-risk boys and 438 early adolescent low-risk boys to a 24-session peer-group intervention administered through local community centers. Feldman's experimental design cleverly varied the groups in several ways, in order to evaluate the impact of therapy group composition (e.g., high-risk boys only, low-risk boys only, or mixed groups), group leader experience, and therapeutic approach (e.g., traditional, behavioral, or minimal). The "traditional social work" intervention group used guided group interaction and group dynamics focused on problem behaviors to elicit insight and commitment to change. The behavioral groups were highly structured attempts to apply group contingencies and systematic reinforcement to improve group behavior. Minimal intervention control groups met, but without a therapeutic goal. Unfortunately, the interventions examined in this effort also proved to be ineffective. Data from direct observations of boys' behavior, self-reports of deviant behavior, and therapist ratings all indicated a disappointingly low impact on boys' outcomes (Feldman et al., 1983). But several interaction effects suggested some ways that future interventions might need to be structured. High-risk boys who were placed in groups together, had inexperienced therapists, and who received process-oriented guidance became increasingly antisocial over time. In contrast, boys in groups run by experienced therapists and following a behavior change agenda fared better.

In addition, when deviant boys were placed with nondeviant peers, their outcomes were more favorable. These findings pointed to the conclusion that high-risk early adolescent boys could be positively affected by being matched with nondeviant peers, with an experienced therapist, using behavior change principles (Feldman et al., 1983).

## DESTINY VERSUS DEVELOPMENTAL ORIENTATIONS

As the crime curve for adolescents continued to rise through the first half of the 1990s, John Dilulio, a political scientist, and James Fox, a sociologist, began to write about a phenomena they described as "super predators." Using the metaphor of wolf packs to describe violent teenagers in a 1995 issue of *The Weekly Standard,* Dilulio predicted that tens of thousands of severely impoverished juvenile super predators were on the near horizon of American culture. This prediction was based (mistakenly, as the findings of the Fast Track study later demonstrate) on an assumption that the 7% of children who account for half of all juvenile crime fit a super-predator profile and could not be deflected from a life of violence. During this same period, the media coverage of juvenile crime framed as part of the super-predator threat led to increasing initiatives to treat juvenile offenders as adults and to focus on incarceration efforts as opposed to treatment alternatives. Incidents such as those mentioned at the outset of this chapter and even more dramatic tragedies such as the Columbine massacre in 1999 resulted in zero tolerance for weapons legislation, making it mandatory to suspend or expel offending youth from schools (Krisberg, 2005). This movement toward getting "tough on crime" led to laws such as "three strikes and you're out" that would keep recidivists in prison for the rest of their lives. The deterministic idea that youth showing early problems were hopeless was fueled by books such as *The Bell Curve* (Herrnstein & Murray, 1994). These authors offered the criticism that "much of public policy toward the disadvantaged starts from the premise that interventions can make up for genetic or environmental disadvantages, and that premise is overly optimistic" (p. 550).

At the same time that these restrictive and nonmalleable orientations toward aggressive children were emerging in the media and reflected in some policies, extensive research was accumulating from the 1970s and 1980s, leading to rapid advancements in the understanding of the developmental processes associated with CD and adolescent delinquency. More detail on this research is described in the following chapter. By the late 1980s and early 1990s, consensus was emerging among researchers that CD rates might be reduced effectively with preventive interventions, with the potential to prevent or substantially reduce later adolescent and adult crime and violence.

It was becoming clear that chronic violence most often emerged when children grew up in high-risk communities and experienced multiple, sequential adversities, including a harsh home life, unstable supports, peer rejection, and academic difficulties. Emerging research suggested that the risk for chronic violence accumulated over time—and the outcomes of at-risk youth might be changed with the right kind of early supports. Longitudinal research conducted by the Oregon Social Learning Center (Patterson, Reid, & Dishion, 1992) had begun to identify a set of specific developmental processes that distinguished children who exhibited antisocial behavior early in childhood and escalated in later adolescence from youth who engaged in delinquency only later, in adolescence.

As described in the following chapter, these developmental studies provided a foundation for the design of the Fast Track program, which was based on the premise that prevention efforts need to begin in childhood, focusing on children with early-starting aggressive behaviors and targeting risk and protective factors identified in developmental research. Fast Track was also supported by a set of short-term prevention and treatment studies that documented how constructed interventions that were grounded in developmental theory could improve parenting and reduce child aggression and promote early competencies.

An important model was provided by the Montreal Prevention Experiment (McCord, Tremblay, Vitaro, & Desmarais-Gervais, 1994). Eighty-four aggressive boys between the ages of 7 and 9 were identified from Montreal schools serving low socioeconomic status (SES), French-speaking families. Half of these boys ($n = 43$) were given an intervention involving 20 sessions of parent training and prosocial skill training across a 2-year period. Rates of self-reported thefts were lower for the intervention group than the control group when youth were evaluated at 10–12 years of age, and self-reported delinquency was similarly significantly lower for intervention youth at 11–15 years of age. However, a report followed the participants into early adulthood (until age 28) and effects on personal violence were no longer significant at that point in time (Vitaro, Brendgen, Giguère, & Tremblay, 2013). One possible implication from these initially promising findings was that a more sustained intervention might have yielded stronger effects.

The substantial research base on the development of CD, along with the short-term benefits associated with small-scale interventions testing parenting or school-based interventions, provided a strong foundation for a more ambitious effort at large-scale prevention. Whereas most interventions targeted a specific factor in the development of the problem, the Montreal Prevention Experiment provided an example of a multicomponent approach. These studies were somewhat encouraging but fell short of providing long-term documentation that prevention of youth violence was possible. As a group, these studies suggested that what was really needed was a large test of a multicomponent, long-term intervention with children who were at high risk for the most serious forms of CD. This was the goal of Fast Track.

In the following chapter, we describe the developmental and intervention research that informed the design of Fast Track in more detail. In subsequent chapters, we describe details of the intervention program and empirical findings about its impact. At the conclusion of this volume, we return to some of the issues raised in this first chapter and discuss the lessons learned from this large and extensive prevention trial.

# Chapter 2

# The Developmental Model
# and Prevention Program Design

The primary aim of the Fast Track project was to develop, implement, and evaluate a comprehensive intervention to prevent the development of CD and related patterns of severe and chronic antisocial and violent behaviors in a sample of children selected as high risk when they first entered elementary school. The intervention was guided by a set of developmental theories that posited the interaction of multiple influences at different developmental periods that influenced child antisocial behavioral development. In this chapter, we summarize research that served as a foundation for us on the development of CD and the difficulties inherent in its prevention, presenting a developmental model of the disorder. We then explore the issues and implications of this developmental model for prevention program design. Although there are now more recent references and findings for many of the ideas we discuss, we write this chapter focusing primarily on our knowledge and reasoning at the time at which we began the project (i.e., 1990) to show its historical perspective.

## EARLY-STARTING CONDUCT PROBLEMS

As noted in Chapter 1, by the early 1990s a consensus had emerged among developmental and clinical researchers that children at high risk for later chronic violence could be identified based on high levels of aggressive conduct problems (Moffitt, 1993; Patterson et al., 1992). A key limitation of this research before 1990 was that it focused almost exclusively on boys, and there was little reliable knowledge about etiology or continuity of CD in girls. In addition, in 1990 it was still unclear how early this developmental trajectory could be identified. Most previous longitudinal studies had begun in middle childhood and there was little careful process research across childhood to elucidate how minor conduct problems in early life (e.g., noncompliance, tantrums, hitting, yelling) became transformed into costly and serious violent behaviors in adolescence. Numerous risk factors had been identified, implicating child temperament, parenting practices, peer relations, and the nature of the school and neighborhood contexts as influences on the developmental processes associated with trajectories of antisocial behavior versus healthy adaptation. It was also recognized that children with the most negative outcomes typically experienced multiple risk factors, creating substantial challenges for the design of an effective prevention program.

In the 1990s (and this is still true today), CD was one of the most intractable mental health problems of childhood and adolescence. Its prevalence today is estimated to range from approximately 4% to 10%, with higher rates in boys than girls. CD is comprised of a cluster of antisocial behaviors, including stealing, lying, running away, physical violence, cruelty, and sexually coercive behavior. This disorder is characterized by frequent conflicts and hostile behavior toward others (parents, teachers, and peers). In adolescence it often includes the perpetration of physical aggression resulting in injury, pain, and property damage to others.

CD commonly begins in early to middle childhood, often emerging first as oppositional defiant disorder (ODD), and then escalating to higher levels of hostile, aggressive, and destructive behaviors. Many aggressive children also show symptoms of attention-deficit/hyperactivity disorder (ADHD), which combined with early aggression places them at heightened risk for poor adolescent and adult outcomes.

Although up to half of the cases of childhood CD remit by adolescence, rarely do adolescent cases of CD or adult cases of antisocial personality disorder (ASPD) begin without warning signs in early childhood (Patterson et al., 1992; Robins, 1978). By 1990, there was some confidence that adolescent CD (and corresponding risk for chronic antisocial and violent behavior) could be predicted reliably from early childhood behavior and related risk factors with relatively low false negative predictions (Loeber, Lahey, & Thomas, 1991; see also results from Fast Track screening analyses in Chapter 3). It was also known that early forms of CD predict later drug abuse, school dropout, suicide, other psychological disorders, and criminality in adolescence and adulthood, suggesting that early prevention might have multiple benefits for individuals and society (Loeber & Dishion, 1983; Robins, 1978; West &

Farrington, 1973). Existing research suggested that CD becomes increasingly resistant to change as children age, in spite of extraordinary efforts in treatment (Kazdin, 1987; McMahon, Wells, & Kotler, 2006), further fueling NIMH's interest in funding studies targeting early intervention and CD prevention.

## INTERVENTIONS TO PREVENT CD IN CHILDREN

Prior to 1990, numerous short-term interventions were directed at young children who showed high rates of aggressive or impulsive behavior. These interventions were based on a variety of theoretical models (behavioral, social-cognitive, and sociological), but generally showed only limited effectiveness (Kazdin, 1987; Lytton, 1990). Several approaches, particularly interventions that targeted parent behavior management strategies and interventions that strengthened the social-cognitive skills and competencies of aggressive children, showed promise in terms of short-term benefits. However, a particular challenge was to produce improvements that generalized across home and school contexts and were sustained across time. Only a few studies had attempted large-scale interventions with long-term follow-up, as reviewed briefly in Chapter 1, and these had not proven effective (although the Montreal Prevention Experiment approach appeared very promising at the time). When Fast Track began, no known study had been successful in the long-term prevention of CD.

When initiating Fast Track, we anticipated that prevention efforts might be strengthened by addressing the following limitations associated with past efforts. First, a clearly articulated developmental model was needed to guide the design of interventions targeting short-term, proximal goals in ways that might lead to long-term impact on future CD. That is, to be successful, intervention efforts should be based strategically on a comprehensive, research-based model of the development of CD. Second and relatedly, we conceptualized CD as a chronic disorder that emerges in a cumulative fashion, aggravated by age-related stressors at key developmental transition points such as school entry and the transition into middle school. Thus, we thought that an effective preventive intervention should continue across developmental periods, with more intensive efforts positioned around these transitional stress points. Third, many past intervention efforts focused on just a single aspect of CD (such as the child's social-cognitive skills or behavioral deficits, or parental discipline practices). Given that CD usually develops in a context of multiple determinants (family stress, parenting deficits, alienation between school and family, child social skill deficits, and academic failure), it is not surprising that single-focus interventions had limited effects. We believed that preventive intervention would be stronger if it was more comprehensive and attentive to the social contexts of the family, peer group, classroom, and neighborhood, as well as the connections between these contexts (e.g., family and school connection). Finally, there was a need to recognize and attend to the heterogeneity among high-risk children. Just as the determinants of CD are multiple, the needs and intervention responsiveness of different individual children and families also vary. As a result, the Fast Track prevention program included both standard components that were implemented consistently for all participating schools, families, and children, and adapted components that provided tailored interventions to address variations in the needs, risks, and competencies of each child and family.

## THE FAST TRACK DEVELOPMENTAL MODEL OF CD

The Fast Track prevention program began with a well-specified developmental model that guided the strategic selection of preventive intervention foci and timing. This developmental model identified key risk and protective factors associated with the course of CD at different developmental periods. In light of the multiple factors associated with the development of CD, the model included child factors, socialization supports (parents, teachers, peers), and contextual influences (family, school, neighborhood) that were implicated in either amplifying or reducing risk for antisocial behavioral development. See Figure 2.1, which provides a graphic overview of the developmental model. Although there are many current references that support such a model, here we reference findings at the time we began the project.

### Early Childhood Years

By 1990, a growing body of research suggested that the precursors of CD often emerge initially during the first several years of life (Campbell, 1991). As early as ages 2 and 3, child characteristics such as irritability and noncompliance along with inattentiveness and impulsivity increase risk for the development of CD in later childhood. These early childhood problems emerge and escalate most often when families are stressed (by poverty, single-parent status, instability), and when parents are distressed, depressed, and harsh in their approach to discipline. Although many factors (including genetics) contribute to early childhood conduct problems, the transactions that occur among family members play a key role in reducing or amplifying child risk for significant conduct problems by the time of formal school entry.

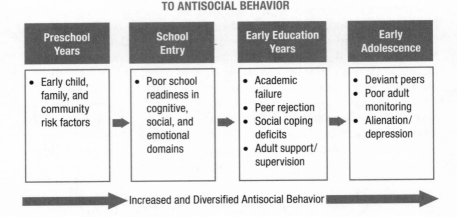

**"EARLY STARTER" PATHWAY
TO ANTISOCIAL BEHAVIOR**

| Preschool Years | School Entry | Early Education Years | Early Adolescence |
|---|---|---|---|
| • Early child, family, and community risk factors | • Poor school readiness in cognitive, social, and emotional domains | • Academic failure<br>• Peer rejection<br>• Social coping deficits<br>• Adult support/ supervision | • Deviant peers<br>• Poor adult monitoring<br>• Alienation/ depression |

Increased and Diversified Antisocial Behavior

**FIGURE 2.1.** Fast Track developmental model.

When Fast Track planning was underway, the most influential short-term developmental model for describing the family dynamics underlying early childhood conduct problems was Patterson's theory of coercive family process (Patterson et al., 1992). In this model, stressful conditions in families (such as financial difficulties, marital conflict and instability, parental disorder, or unpreparedness for parenting) make it difficult for parents to set limits consistently for their children or provide effective positive behavioral support for them, especially when the children themselves have characteristics such as temperamental irritability or impulsivity. Without effective guidance, children can become increasingly noncompliant, aggressive, and impulsive. According to the theory, an escalating cycle of aversive exchanges with parents emerges in which children learn to respond to requests for compliance with negative, resistant verbalizations and behavior. When beleaguered parents give in to such behavior or give up their attempts to gain compliance, they promote the likelihood of increasingly aversive and hostile child behavior on future occasions. In this way, children develop the skilled use of aversive behavior in social interactions. Increasing parental demoralization accompanies this cycle, and parents often withdraw or alienate themselves from their outside sources of social support, thus adding stress to the family system.

In addition to the negative behavioral impact of coercive parent–child interactions, these relationship dynamics also undermine healthy emotional development. Frequent parent–child conflict and unpredictable (sometimes frightening) threats and punishment weaken the parent–child attachment that serves as a core foundation for developing emotional well-being (Greenberg, Kusché, & Speltz, 1991). In addition, parent–child conflict is often accompanied by low levels of parental stimulation and lack of support for the child's development of positive self-regulation, emotional control, and social skills. Developing the capacity to manage strong emotions effectively requires an integration of affect, language, cognition, and action (Greenberg et al., 1991). That is, young children need to learn to recognize internal cues of affect, to label them with appropriate terms, and to develop cognitive skills for self-monitoring in order to translate strong negative feelings into socially adaptive behavior. Parents who react to negative expressions of child affect as being intolerable or frightening not only involve their children in coercive cycles of aversive interpersonal control, but also fail to assist them in developing internalized forms of control or appropriate expressions of these emotions.

Finally, children with CD often receive poor cognitive stimulation and support from their parents, which may contribute to low levels of academic readiness at school entry. Concurrent child problems of inattentiveness and hyperactivity may also impede children's readiness as they transition into school (Campbell, 1991; Moffitt, 1993).

## Middle Childhood Years

During elementary school, negative school and peer experiences can further exacerbate the adjustment difficulties of children with conduct problems.

When children enter school with deficits in key areas of self-regulation and social competence, they struggle to establish positive relationships with teachers and peers. Associated problems of inattention and hyperactivity often contribute to early learning difficulties and further exacerbate early social-emotional deficits. When children carry over their noncompliant and aggressive behaviors into the school setting, they elicit censure from teachers and peers. Teachers often report an inability to develop the trusting relationship that is especially necessary to support child attention and motivation for learning. Across time, peers become increasingly wary and avoidant of these children and they become rejected and, in some cases, excluded and victimized by peers. A key consequence is that these children miss out on many of the normal, positive peer experiences experienced by most children in school that support positive social-emotional development. The lack of important social skills, including the ability to manage strong feelings, resolve conflicts, and communicate effectively, contributes to a negative cycle of rejection, social exclusion, and lack of positive developmental support. Ostracized by better-adjusted classmates, aggressive children tend to befriend one another, increasing exposure to negative peer influence (Coie, 1990).

As a consequence of early conflicts with parents, along with exposure to hostile peer relations, aggressive elementary school children begin to display biases in their social perceptions and social reasoning (Dodge, Bates, & Pettit, 1990). Relative to their peers, aggressive children often fail to attend to relevant social cues, inaccurately interpret peers' intentions, and presume hostile intent in ambiguous situations. They are often unskilled in social problem solving, displaying an impoverished repertoire of competent verbally assertive strategies, and instead showing a tendency to access action-oriented and aggressive responses. They also are more likely than their nonaggressive classmates to evaluate aggression as leading to positive interpersonal and instrumental outcomes. Dodge and colleagues reported that these biases are predictable from early family experiences, such as overly harsh discipline practices, and they lead to the later development of social and behavioral difficulties in school. Moreover, these biases and deficits mediate the effect of early family experiences on later conduct problems, providing a link between early experiences and later CD.

Several consequences follow from this spiraling pattern of child aversive behavior, interpersonal rejection, and negative reactivity that characterizes the development of chronically aggressive children during middle childhood. One is that high-risk children perform poorly in school and become alienated from the goals and values of this major socializing institution. A second consequence is that some of these children become depressed and develop negative self-concepts in cognitive, social, and behavioral domains. A third consequence is that rejected, aggressive children often drift into deviant peer groups in early adolescence, feeling alienated from mainstream peers and social institutions (Coie, 1990).

## Middle School and High School Years

Early adolescence is marked both by changes in the youth's own characteristics as well as in the contextual influences affecting adjustment. Contextually, youth move from self-contained, single-teacher elementary classrooms to large, fluid middle or junior high schools (Eccles, Midgley, & Adler, 1984), with corresponding reductions in parent and teacher support and monitoring. Consequently, youth spend more time with, and are more influenced by, their peers.

By early adolescence, alienation from the mainstream culture and association with deviant peers play a particularly critical role in promoting adolescent delinquency. Peer rejection and aggression in middle childhood are predictive of deviant group membership in early adolescence, about the time of transition from elementary school to middle school (Dishion & Tipsord, 2011). Peer rejection and aggression in the elementary years are also significantly predictive of CD in the first year of middle school (Coie, Lochman, Terry, & Hyman, 1992). Connection and identification with the deviant peer group in adolescence is a key potentiating context for delinquency, early substance abuse, and early, risky sex. Adolescents who associate with deviant peers have a substantially increased risk for adolescent problem behaviors and adolescent arrest (Coie et al., 1992). Keenan and colleagues found that, in comparison to boys who did not have best friends who were truant or disobedient, disruptive boys who had deviant peer associations were three to four times more likely to participate in covert and overt delinquent acts (Keenan, Loeber, Zhang, Stouthamer-Loeber, & Van Kammen, 1995). Within deviant peer groups, adolescents reinforce each other's antisocial beliefs and attitudes. Deviant peer influences serve both to instigate initial delinquency among those with marginal risk profiles and to escalate the seriousness of offending among youth with a history of delinquency (Thornberry, 1987).

Whereas girls are at considerably lower risk than boys for overt aggression during elementary school, their risk for becoming involved in early sexual activity, substance use, and covert antisocial activity rises in adolescence, due largely to associations with older antisocial boys (Caspi, Lynam, Moffitt, & Silva, 1993). Girls who enter puberty early and who have learning problems and depressed mood are at elevated risk for associations with older delinquent boys who, in turn, encourage behaviors such as truancy, substance use, covert delinquency, and sexual activity.

In addition to deviant peer affiliations, low levels of school engagement also place young adolescents at risk for escalating problem behaviors (Hawkins & Weiss, 1995). Adolescents who dislike school and spend little time on homework are frequently truant, show poor achievement, and have high rates of drug use. Increasing school adaptation by fostering social support in the school setting, promoting positive attitudes toward education, and supporting academic achievement may avoid adolescents' declines in school attachment and self-esteem and reduce negative outcomes such as early initiation of sexual activity.

Adolescents' rates of problem behaviors are also heavily influenced by their deviance-prone attitudes and beliefs, including undervaluing school attendance and academic achievement along with a high tolerance for deviant behaviors such as stealing and lying. Adolescents with histories of conduct problems are often impulsive and emotionally reactive, and they often show hostile attributional biases and dominance-oriented social goals, combined with poor self-control and weak social problem-solving skills. As adolescents become increasingly autonomous and as demands for self-discipline increase in schoolwork and other areas, these social-cognitive biases, attitudes, and skill deficits increase risk for school failure and promote school disengagement and antisocial activity. School seems worthless and boring, whereas antisocial activity appears rewarding and enjoyable.

At the same time, for some adolescents, especially in certain minority groups, subcultural values and expectations make it difficult to attain certain positive goals, such as achieving school success. Socially marked identities, such as being a black male, can make adolescents vulnerable to failure because of stereotype threat vulnerability—expectations of failure that the youth contends with as he or she learns and performs (Steele & Aronson, 1995). Contending with these negative expectations or stereotypes can undermine achievement. Thus, many black males, for example, may not pursue academic success because these identities carry with them the shared expectation that academic failure is unavoidable, and because their peers do not seem to value school success.

This cascade of events that can occur during middle and high school to promote antisocial development is further potentiated by inadequate parental monitoring at home. As aggressive children get older, they tend to withdraw from their parents, and their parents tend to withdraw from them (Patterson et al., 1992). Years of coercive interactions train parents and children to avoid conflict with the other. As a result, parents may increasingly fail to monitor their children's activities, and children are left unsupervised to engage in delinquent behaviors. Parents may have negative encounters with teachers about their children's school-based behaviors, which, coupled with continued and escalating aversive interactions with their children in the home, lead some parents to reject their highly aggressive children and show less interest in them as they enter adolescence. Because of the greater mobility of adolescents and their increased needs for personal privacy, parents have less opportunity to monitor their adolescents' activities and their friendships, and their knowledge about youth activities rests heavily on youths' willingness to disclose this information (Kerr & Stattin, 2000). Research indicates that poor parental monitoring and discipline play a critical role in adolescents' involvement in deviant peer groups, and in early- and late-onset delinquency and drug use (Racz & McMahon, 2011).

## THE ROLE OF CONTEXT AND RISK

In addition to a developmental model that can guide intervention in addressing pathways to CD, an ecological framework is also necessary to fully represent the influences affecting the development of CD. Bronfenbrenner (1979) had elucidated the importance of multiple levels of influence on child development, including proximal influences by interactions with family members, peers, and teachers (i.e., microsystem) and contextual factors that operate at the level of the school and neighborhood (i.e., exosystem). At the community level, living in a poor, crime-ridden neighborhood with low rates of employment, having relatively few support services and community resources for parents, and having parents who are isolated and disconnected from helpful social supports all increase child risk for developing CD. These community-level factors contribute directly by increasing child exposure to risky models and high stress levels, and they contribute indirectly, by undermining parenting capacity (Greenberg, Lengua, Coie, Pinderhughes, & CPPRG, 1999).

During the elementary school years, the school context can also become an exacerbating rather than a corrective influence shaping child development. More often than not, high-risk children attend schools in which there is a high density of other high-risk children, creating an atmosphere less conducive to learning and more evocative of CD. This, in turn, makes teaching more difficult and, for inexperienced or highly stressed teachers, can lead to a reenactment of the coercive and inconsistent home situation in the classroom context. Furthermore, schools in poor and high-crime neighborhoods have a high rate of poorly prepared and inadequately resourced teachers. Such schools are allocated and spend substantially fewer dollars per child, have high teacher turnover, and high rates of student dropout.

## IMPLICATIONS OF THE DEVELOPMENTAL MODEL
## FOR INTERVENTION

Because children at high risk for CD are likely to progress in a spiral of escalating and more severe conduct problems over time, early intervention is critical. Over time, these children become increasingly enmeshed in accumulating risk factors, with peer rejection and academic failure adding to parent–child conflict, complicating the ease and effectiveness of intervention. In addition, the developmental process is dynamic, such that risk markers change with age. Early risk factors influence subsequent developmental processes within the child and the family, increasing exposure to negative socialization experiences, which further compound the child's risk for ultimate antisocial outcomes.

The dysfunctional development that is associated with the early-starting pattern of conduct problems is multiply determined, involving transactions among child characteristics and family, peer, school, and neighborhood influences. Accordingly, prevention efforts must target both the promotion of individual competencies that can serve as protective factors and the promotion of protective contextual supports. Preventive interventions must also be attentive to age-related stressors and the successive issues of risk that emerge at school entry and during the transition into adolescence.

This comprehensive developmental model suggests two strategic points in childhood for preventive intervention (CPPRG, 1992, 2000). First, by school entry there is an identifiable constellation of child and family variables that indicate high risk for emerging and escalating CD. Because school entry is a significant developmental transition, and failure has not yet occurred, families may be hopeful and motivated to support their child's school success. In addition, during developmental transitions, families are both under more stress and often more open to learning new skills, which may foster responsiveness to proactive interventions such as Fast Track.

In designing the Fast Track intervention, we conceptualized six interrelated short-term targets for elementary school prevention, following from the developmental model (shown in Figure 2.2). First, high-risk children need help in learning to control anger, in developing social-cognitive skills, and in generating more socially acceptable and effective alternatives to aggression and oppositional behavior. Second, in addition to these coping skills, aggressive children need guided, controlled

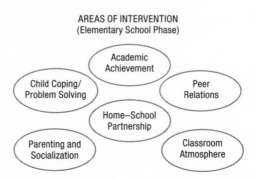

**FIGURE 2.2.** Interrelated targets of the early elementary phase intervention.

experiences that facilitate the development of friendships that are pro-social and that demonstrate caring and concern for others. Third, many high-risk children need concentrated assistance in preparing for the academic tasks of school, most especially early reading. Fourth, their parents need to acquire more consistent, more positive, and less punitive discipline methods; to learn how to better regulate their own emotions during conflict; and to learn how to provide support for their children's cognitive growth. Fifth, many parents need support in learning to relate to teachers and to provide support at home for the school's goals for their children (e.g., effective home–school partnership). Sixth, teachers may need help in preparing their classrooms with effective and caring atmo-spheres that support healthy social development and learning for all chil-dren, especially in schools and classrooms with a high concentration of high-risk children. In Fast Track, we hypothesized that improving the quality of the school and classroom climate and facilitating positive child "bonding" to both family and school as well as the family's posi-tive connection to the school and other social institutions could serve as important protective factors for school success and the prevention of CD.

As described in more detail in Chapter 4, the Fast Track elemen-tary school intervention based upon this developmental model included an integrated set of intervention components to promote competencies in children (social-emotional skills training and academic tutoring), parents (parent management training and home visiting), and teachers (prevention curriculum and classroom management consultation), and to strengthen bonds of communication between parents and teachers. Given our conceptual model, one goal was to promote a more positive school environment for all children as well as building the social and social-cognitive skills of high-risk aggressive children. For this reason, the Fast Track intervention featured a classroom-level (universal) inter-vention component, as well as components specifically for the high-risk children and their families (targeted interventions). We hypothesized reciprocal benefits for these universal and targeted interventions. As classroom climate improves as a function of the classroom-level inter-vention and teacher consultation, it should promote a more positive socializing environment for the high-risk children, thus facilitating more appropriate behavior and attitudes. Conversely, as the targeted inter-vention components affect the high-risk group, these children will be less disruptive in the classroom and less aggressive on the playground, enhancing the classroom climate and corresponding learning and social opportunities of all children.

Although the negative impact of early risk factors may be buffered by the provision of protective support services during the grade school years, the risk factors themselves may continue to influence developmental trajectories during adolescence. For example, the high rates of inattention, impulsivity, and cognitive deficits that contribute to the school adjustment problems of many early-starting youth (Moffitt, 1993) may be buffered when protective support is offered during elementary school in the form of academic tutoring and effective teacher management. As the demands for focused attention and independent work completion increase with the transition to middle school, however, these cognitive risk factors may undermine school adaptation unless continuing support is offered at these later grade levels. In addition, developmental research suggests that new risk factors (e.g., antisocial peers, neurological changes leading to greater impulsivity and risk taking) emerge during adolescence that are associated with the escalation of antisocial and related adolescent behavior problems. Elementary school prevention may improve child "readiness" to tackle the new challenges of adolescence. However, for high-risk children living in unstable and risky contexts, additional protective supports may be needed during the transition into adolescence to sustain the gains produced by early preventive efforts. Thus, a successful program for preventing serious antisocial problems may require a long-term intervention commitment, targeting multiple domains.

Hence, a second logical point for intervention is at the transition into middle school, where key issues include the control of aggressive and disruptive behavior, the acquisition and use of prosocial skills for integrating into the mainstream peer culture, and concentrated assistance with academic skills. Youth may also profit from individual competency-enhancing experiences related to their own developing goals and interests (both in and outside of school) to maintain or restore self-esteem and positive expectations for success. Adolescents' "possible selves" (i.e., their images of who they would strive to be) serve to guide their choices and are important motivators of behavior (Markus & Nurias, 1986; Oyserman & Markus, 1993). Among high-risk youth, resilient adolescents are those who develop a positive sense of self, perceive themselves to have internal control over their environment, develop a sense of purpose, and have good problem-solving skills and a strong network of relationships with adults. Indeed, interventions that combine training in social-influence resistance with problem solving and decision making have produced reductions in the prevalence of substance use (Botvin, 1986; Hansen, Graham, Wolkenstein, & Lundy, 1988). The availability of a positive adult role model and mentor who is of the same race and gender as the high-risk youth may also serve as a protective factor promoting the development of a positive sense of self/identity and supporting effective coping skills (Dubois & Karcher, 2006). In addition, parents of high-risk adolescents need to establish effective and nonpunitive limit setting and maintain or regain an active interest in their activities so that reasonable monitoring of adolescent behavior can occur. Productive parent–adolescent communication, joint problem solving, and collaborative planning are all indices of supportive family relations in adolescence; interventions focused on promoting communication and conflict resolution skills along with family problem-solving meetings reduce adolescent acting-out behaviors (Henggeler, Schoenwald, & Pickrel, 1995). Effective parental monitoring works both directly to promote more positive adolescent behavior, and indirectly by protecting adolescents from involvement in high-risk peer groups. Furthermore, some active partnership between parents and schools must take place if the monitoring of homework, school attendance, and resistance to deviant peer group involvement is to take place.

## SUMMARY

The significance of the Fast Track project is that it addressed three organizing principles for the prevention of serious violent delinquency outlined by Thornberry, Huizinga, and Loeber (1995): (1) it started early, (2) it was comprehensive, and (3) it was carried out over the long term of development. In Fast Track, high-risk youth were selected at school entry from poor, transient, high-crime neighborhoods. A fundamental premise of the Fast Track model was that, in most cases, serious CD emerges as part of an escalating early-starting cycle that reflects both individual factors (e.g., affect regulation, cognitive reasoning) and socialization influences (e.g., increasing conflicts with parents, teachers, and peers; ineffective supervision and limit setting by parents). This constellation of individual and socialization factors is especially detrimental in high-stress, low-resource neighborhoods, which increase exposure to threat and reduce available social support.

As we conceived of the model in 1990, the Fast Track developmental model of CD suggested a prevention strategy that encompassed the first 6 or 7 years of schooling for high-risk children, with particularly intensive interventions during the transitions at school entry and at the entrance to middle school. As the study progressed, we also came to believe it was important to intervene through the transition to high school as well. In light of the many and pervasive factors operating to promote antisocial tendencies among high-risk children, we anticipated that only a comprehensive, long-term, and multicomponent prevention design could have a pronounced effect on the incidence of CD, delinquency, adolescent violence, and related problems in this population.

# Chapter 3

# Project Design, Sample, and Screening

In this chapter, we describe the study design and the children and families who participated in Fast Track. The overall goal of Fast Track was to evaluate the effectiveness of a multiyear prevention program for children identified as high risk for developing CD based on elevated aggression in kindergarten. Although Fast Track included a universal prevention component provided to all children (i.e., the PATHS® [Promoting Alternative Thinking Strategies] curriculum; Kusché, Greenberg, & CPPRG, 2011), all other prevention components were designed for delivery at the indicated level of prevention—provided only to those children who were identified as showing early signs of developing CD and intended to prevent development of the full-blown disorder (Mrazek et al., 1994). For serious but low base-rate problems such as future antisocial violence, we assumed that an indicated prevention program was preferable because it can be more focused, more efficient, and more intensive than a universal preventive intervention (Lochman & CPPRG, 1995; Offord, 2000). However, the lower the base rate of a condition, the greater the need for accuracy in screening. Potential savings of time, money, and other resources offered by an indicated intervention represent true savings only to the extent that the intervention is effective, delivered to those who truly need it, and not delivered to those who do not need it (Hill, Lochman, & CPPRG, 2004). Hence, the first step in the Fast Track process was the application of a screening and selection process to identify high-risk children in kindergarten, along with a randomization process to define the intervention and control groups. This chapter provides an overview of these processes and a description of the resulting sample. We also provide data on the predictive validity of the screening system and data on sample retention over time. Finally, we introduce two case studies that we share in subsequent chapters to illustrate differences in how youth and families engaged with Fast Track and progressed over time.

## SCREENING PROCESSES AND SAMPLE SELECTION

The Fast Track trial involved the application of similar procedures at four geographically diverse sites. The sites represented a range of urban settings (Nashville, TN; Durham, NC; Seattle, WA) and a rural setting (three rural communities within 1 hour of State College, PA), providing the capacity to assess the generalizability of findings in different contexts. These sites were located near the universities of the Fast Track principal investigators, which allowed the prevention research teams to closely monitor and support the high-fidelity implementation of the prevention program and collect extensive developmental data.

As a first step to identifying high-risk children, we selected 52 elementary schools within these sites (13 schools in Durham, NC; 7 in Nashville, TN; 16 in Seattle, WA; and 16 in rural central Pennsylvania) as "high risk" based on crime and poverty statistics of the neighborhoods that they served. Three additional schools in Nashville that served kindergarten children who entered participating elementary schools were also included in the screening process, producing a total of 55 schools across all four sites participating in screening. The characteristics of these schools varied across the four sites: Durham (90% ethnic minority, 80% of students qualifying for free/reduced-price lunch); Nashville (54% ethnic minority, 78% free/reduced-price lunch); Seattle (52% ethnic minority, 45% free/reduced-price lunch); and rural central Pennsylvania (1% ethnic minority, 39% free/reduced-price lunch).

Several considerations informed the screening processes. First, we decided to conduct the screening when children were in kindergarten. This timing was based on a desire to identify samples of high-risk children who were representative of those in the four respective communities; timing the screening after school entry increased the likelihood of a full population-based screen. In addition, timing the intervention at the start of elementary school allowed us to frame the intervention as an opportunity for parents to help their children make the best start possible in school. Our goal was to start the prevention program as soon as possible once the children entered school to help prevent the negative cascade that often occurs after aggressive children enter school and experience social and academic difficulties. We thus focused on early winter in the kindergarten year to initiate screening, so that teachers would know their children well.

Second, we chose to focus on children's aggressive behavior as a basis for the screening based on longitudinal studies linking early aggression with later CD and antisocial behavior (see Chapters 1 and 2). We considered including other risk factors in the screening process, especially problematic parenting practices, as well as poverty and single-parent status, given that they may amplify child risks. In the screening of the first cohort, we included a measure of problematic parenting practices, but found that it was redundant with the behavioral ratings of risk, and did not contribute additional information toward high-risk designation. Consequently we dropped it with subsequent cohorts. As planned, there were a total of three annual cohorts.

A third decision focused on the method used to assess children's early conduct problems. We decided to avoid cumbersome and expensive measurement strategies that could not be scaled up effectively, such as direct observation of child behavior and peer-rated sociometric procedures. Instead, we focused on teachers and parents as informants, reasoning that they would be both knowledgeable about the child and accessible. We felt that each source had unique advantages, and so a screener that combined their strengths would be optimal. Teachers have the benefit of being able to rate children's behavior in a relative way, comparing a given child to others of similar age. Parents have the advantage of knowing about their children's functioning outside of the school setting and over time.

Based on these considerations, the identification of students at high risk for antisocial outcomes proceeded in the same way across all schools, with the application of a multiple-gating screening procedure that combined teacher and parent ratings of aggressive and disruptive behaviors (Lochman & CPPRG, 1995). All 9,594 kindergartners across three cohorts (1991–1993) in the 55 participating schools were screened initially by teachers, using the Teacher Observation of Classroom Adaptation—Revised (TOCA-R) Authority Acceptance Scale (Werthamer-Larsson, Kellam, & Wheeler, 1991). On this 10-item measure, teachers rated the degree to which each child in the classroom exhibited aggressive and noncompliant behavior (e.g., fights, breaks rules, is mean to others). Children scoring in the top 40% within each cohort and site were then solicited for the next stage of screening for home behavior problems by the parents, using items from the Child Behavior Checklist (CBCL; Achenbach, 1991a) and similar scales, and 91% agreed ($n = 3,545$). The teacher and parent screen scores were then standardized and combined into a sum score representing a total *severity-of-risk screen score*.

High-risk children were selected for inclusion into the study based on this screen score. Within each of the 24 site-by-cohort-by-condition groups, selection moved from the highest score downward until desired sample sizes were reached. Across the full high-risk sample, 94.4% were in the top 20% of the screen score distribution. Deviations were made when a child failed to matriculate in the first grade at a core school ($n$ = 59) or refused to participate ($n$ = 75), or to accommodate a rule that no child would be the only girl in a friendship intervention group (i.e., Friendship Groups would have no girls or at least two girls). Children were also excluded from the sample if the parents did not speak English, if the children were currently in foster care, or if the families planned to move out of the area within 1 year.

Within each site, the schools were divided into one to three paired sets of schools, matched for demographics (number of students, percentage of children receiving free or reduced lunch, ethnic composition), and one set in each pair was randomly assigned to intervention and one set to the control condition. Randomization occurred at the level of the school cluster to accommodate the decision to implement a universal prevention program, the PATHS curriculum (Kusché et al., 2011), which was taught by classroom teachers to all students. Given this school-level intervention, randomization at the level of the child would lead to contamination of conditions, with some children in the control group receiving this intervention component. One school in Seattle withdrew after randomization to intervention, leaving 54 participating schools. Several years after the start of the Fast Track project, the Durham school district underwent a major reorganization, resulting in the reassignment of students across intervention and control schools and leading us to move the implementation of PATHS outside of the school (described in more detail in Chapter 4).

Across all of these schools, children were recruited in three annual cohorts, starting intervention for the first cohort in fall of 1991, resulting in a total high-risk sample of 891 children. Over time, some children moved from an intervention school kindergarten to a control school (or vice versa). Children were assigned to the intervention or control group based on the school they attended in the fall of their first grade, when the intervention was initiated ($n$'s = 445 for intervention and 446 for control).

In terms of problem levels, the average kindergarten externalizing $T$ score on the Teacher's Report Form (TRF) of the CBCL (Achenbach, 1991b), which provides national norms (available for 88% of the high-risk sample) was 66.4 (national $M$ = 50; $SD$ = 10), and 76% of the children in the high-risk sample scored in the clinical or subclinical range ($T$ scores of 60 or higher). The mean age of participants was 6.5 years ($SD$

= 0.48) at the time of identification. Across all sites, the sample was primarily composed of black (51%) and white (47%) participants, with 2% of other ethnicity (e.g., Pacific Islander and Hispanic); 69% were boys. The distribution of the sample by sex, race, site, and intervention status is shown in Table 3.1 (CPPRG, 2010b). The sample was skewed toward socioeconomic disadvantage: 58% were from single-parent families, 29% of parents had not completed high school, and 40% of the families were in the lowest socioeconomic class (representing unskilled workers) as scored by Hollingshead (1975). Some differences in distributions were observed within sites. In the sets of schools that were randomized to intervention versus control status in Nashville, schools assigned to the intervention condition included more black children, whereas schools assigned to the control group included more white children. Correspondingly, in Nashville, the intervention group had a higher proportion of black children than the control group (73% vs. 56%). Otherwise, the intervention and control groups were well balanced on race and sex.

In addition to this high-risk sample, we identified a stratified normative sample of 387 children from the 27 control schools in cohort 1 to represent the normative range of risk scores in the participating communities based on teacher ratings of behavior. We followed these children and families for the entire study period so that outcomes for

**TABLE 3.1. Sample by Sex, Race, Site, and Intervention Status**

| | Number of participants | | | | | |
| | Black | | | Non-black | | |
| | Intervention | Control | Norm | Intervention | Control | Norm |
|---|---|---|---|---|---|---|
| Boys | | | | | | |
| Durham | 82 | 75 | 44 | 7 | 4 | 6 |
| Nashville | 64 | 39 | 24 | 22 | 33 | 25 |
| Pennsylvania | 2 | 1 | 1 | 76 | 70 | 48 |
| Seattle | 31 | 29 | 20 | 38 | 45 | 29 |
| Girls | | | | | | |
| Durham | 19 | 27 | 43 | 2 | 3 | 7 |
| Nashville | 19 | 26 | 24 | 9 | 18 | 27 |
| Pennsylvania | 1 | 2 | 0 | 34 | 39 | 49 |
| Seattle | 18 | 17 | 12 | 21 | 18 | 28 |
| Total | 236 | 216 | 168 | 209 | 230 | 219 |

*Note.* Pennsylvania, rural Pennsylvania; Norm, normative sample. Data from CPPRG (2010b).

the intervention group could be contrasted not only with the high-risk control group, but also with those of the normative sample to determine whether they reached normative rates of functioning for their communities. This normative sample also provided the opportunity to study processes of risk and protective factors related to youths' problematic outcomes across time without any confound with the intervention. The normative sample represented the population at the control schools and thus overlapped with the high-risk sample at the upper end of the risk distribution. Across the four sites, 79 students who were identified as high-risk control group participants also were selected to be part of this normative sample of 387. Of the normative sample, 35% came from single-parent families, 23% of mothers had not graduated from high school, 50% were male, and 43% were black.

## DATA COLLECTION PROCESSES

Participants who were screened into the high-risk sample or were randomly selected for the normative sample were formally recruited into the longitudinal study during the summer before children began first grade. That summer and each summer thereafter through the end of high school, parents and children were visited in their home for assessments. Youth were also assessed in the two years after the end of the high school years. While one research assistant interviewed the primary caregiver (usually the mother), a second assistant interviewed the child in a separate room. Interviewers read the various measures to the primary caregivers or children and recorded their responses. In addition, teacher surveys were collected in the spring of each school year and additional data were collected during selected years. For example, classroom observations were collected in first and second grade, peer sociometric ratings were collected in first through fourth grades, and parent–child interactions were observed in the home at kindergarten and first, second, fifth, and eighth grades. After high school, youth interviews were conducted at ages 19, 20, and 25. Throughout the study, interviewers were blind to the participants' intervention status. Beginning in early adolescence, juvenile court records were collected, as were adult court records through age 25. Active parent consent and, at older ages, youth assent (or consent after age 18) was obtained each year, and participants were paid for completing interviews. All procedures were approved by the institutional review boards of participating universities.

Multiple strategies were employed to avoid attrition, and despite the unstable lives of many of the participating families, attrition was fairly low, typically averaging 2–3% per year. For example, 11% of intervention children and 16% of control children did not participate in the follow-up interview by grade 8 (CPPRG, 2010a). By grade 12, 26% of intervention youth and 29% of control youth did not participate in the follow-up interview (CPPRG, 2010b). Figure 3.1 provides a CON-SORT flow chart that indicates the retention of the sample through the end of high school (CPPRG, 2010b). The participation rate for data collection by age 25 improved and was 81% (CPPRG, 2015). There were no differences in attrition by baseline demographics (sex, race) or study variables (condition, cohort) in the high-risk sample by 12th grade (Wu, Witkiewitz, McMahon, Dodge, & CPPRG, 2010). Multiple imputation methods were used to manage missing data in longitudinal analyses.

Across the 29 years of the study to date, a wide range of measures was collected using multi-informant and multimethod strategies. A complete listing of measures, technical reports for measures, and copies of publicly available instruments collected within the Fast Track project are posted at *www.fasttrackproject.org.* In order to account for the heterogeneity of the participants and provide more precise estimates of intervention effects, a set of 19 baseline variables were included as covariates.

Table 3.2 presents data on intervention and control groups for these 19 baseline variables. On most baseline variables, the intervention and control groups were equivalent, including parent daily reports of aggression, teacher TOCA-R screen scores, family SES, primary caregiver mental well-being (e.g., depressive symptoms, social support satisfaction), stressful life events, neighborhood safety, child IQ, child social cognitions (hostile attributions, aggressive retaliation, social problem-solving skills, emotional understanding) and parent-reported appropriate and verbal punishment. Relative to the control group, the intervention group had significantly higher scores on parent-rated social competence and child reading readiness and parents reported less use of physical punishment (CPPRG, 2010a). We conducted additional tests to compare intervention and control groups within subgroups at highest and moderate risk, and did not find any systematic bias between the intervention and control groups. Thus, the randomization process was successful at creating intervention and control groups that were equivalent on almost every baseline variable.

## ACCURACY OF SCREENING THROUGH ELEMENTARY SCHOOL

The function of a screening procedure is to classify individuals into two groups: those who are at greater risk and more likely to develop a problematic outcome (in this case, criminal convictions or other form of antisocial behavior) and those who are not. The test of screening accuracy

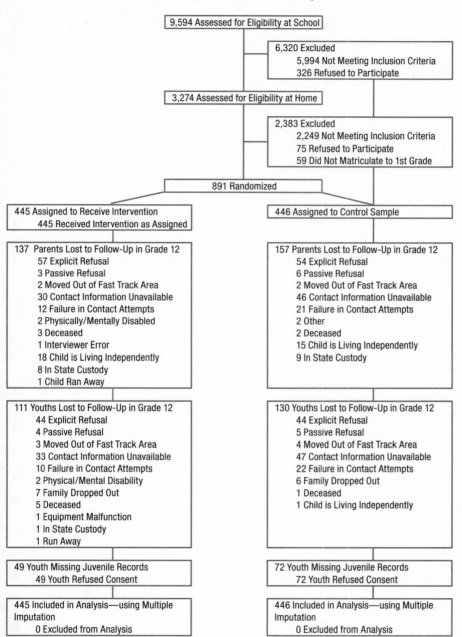

**FIGURE 3.1.** CONSORT flow chart showing participant flow through the end of high school.

**TABLE 3.2. Preintervention Means, Standard Deviations, and Differences across Conditions for Variables That Were Used as Covariates**

| Variable | Range | Intervention | | Control | | df | t | p |
|---|---|---|---|---|---|---|---|---|
| | | M | SD | M | SD | | | |
| Child baseline behavior problems | | | | | | | | |
| Oppositional + aggressive behaviors [PDR] (P) | 0–0.8 | 0.26 | 0.17 | 0.27 | 0.17 | 886 | 0.84 | .40 |
| Authority acceptance [TOCA–R] (T) | 0–5 | 2.18 | 0.95 | 2.24 | 0.96 | 883 | 0.93 | .35 |
| Family demographics and social ecology | | | | | | | | |
| Socioeconomic status (P) | 4–66 | 24.58 | 12.91 | 24.17 | 12.46 | 886 | −0.48 | .63 |
| Maternal depression [CES–D] (P) | 0–57 | 15.83 | 9.84 | 16.81 | 10.42 | 888 | 1.43 | .15 |
| Family satisfaction (P) | 0–3 | 2.11 | 0.76 | 2.18 | 0.68 | 882 | 1.5 | .13 |
| Friendship satisfaction (P) | 0–3 | 2.30 | 0.65 | 2.37 | 0.57 | 885 | 1.83 | .07 |
| Stressful life events scale (P) | 0–24 | 5.25 | 4.24 | 5.3 | 3.97 | 882 | 0.17 | .87 |
| Neighborhood dangerousness rating | −2–1.5 | −0.05 | 0.61 | −0.03 | 0.59 | 888 | 0.51 | .61 |
| Child cognitive and social skills | | | | | | | | |
| IQ [WISC] standardized score (D) | −2.4–3.1 | −0.04 | 0.8 | −0.11 | 0.78 | 887 | −1.18 | .24 |
| Hostile attributional bias (D) | 0–1 | 0.67 | 0.25 | 0.67 | 0.25 | 888 | −0.24 | .81 |
| Aggressive responses to provocation (D) | 0–40 | 22.57 | 8.29 | 22.14 | 8.1 | 886 | −0.79 | .43 |
| Emotion understanding (D) | 0–4 | 3.58 | 0.72 | 3.55 | 0.8 | 889 | −0.51 | .61 |
| Social competence (P) | 0–3.75 | 2.09 | 0.59 | 2.0 | 0.58 | 888 | −2.45 | .01 |
| Letter word identification (D) | 0–40 | 13.05 | 4.98 | 12.18 | 4.01 | 887 | −2.84 | .05 |
| Emotional recognition (D) | 2–16 | 10.73 | 2.77 | 10.69 | 2.84 | 875 | −0.21 | .84 |

**TABLE 3.2** *(continued)*

| Variable | Range | Intervention M | Intervention SD | Control M | Control SD | df | t | p |
|---|---|---|---|---|---|---|---|---|
| | | Parenting behavior | | | | | | |
| Appropriate discipline (P) | 1.1–2.8 | 2.01 | 0.28 | 1.99 | 0.28 | 883 | −0.79 | .43 |
| Physical punishment (P) | 0–1.67 | 0.21 | 0.22 | 0.24 | 0.24 | 887 | 2.17 | .03 |
| Verbal punishment (P) | 0–2 | 0.25 | 0.32 | 0.27 | 0.31 | 887 | 1.03 | .30 |
| Warmth toward child (O) | 1.1–5 | 3.62 | 0.8 | 3.54 | 0.78 | 886 | −1.55 | .12 |

*Note.* Instruments are described in detail at *www.fasttrackproject.org*. P, parent rating; T, teacher rating; D, direct assessment; O, observer rating; CES-D, Center for Epidemiological Studies Depression Scale; PDR, Parent Daily Report; TOCA-R, Teacher Observation of Classroom Adaptation—Revised; WISC, Weschler Intelligence Scale for Children. Data from CPPRG (2010a).

is based on the association of this risk classification with classification on another binary outcome: those who have developed CD or related antisocial behaviors and those who have not (Hill et al., 2004). Statistics that test a screen's accuracy are derived from the matrix of these two binary outcomes and include *sensitivity* (the proportion of true positives correctly identified); *specificity* (the proportion of true negatives correctly identified); *positive predictive value* (PPV, the proportion of those classified as at risk who developed the problematic outcome); and *negative predictive value* (NPV, the proportion classified as not at risk in whom the problematic outcome is absent). Generally speaking, when the cut point of a screen is set at a lower threshold (e.g., less risk is needed to enter the high-risk group), there are fewer false positives and therefore greater sensitivity, but there are also more false negatives, and therefore lower specificity. Greater sensitivity is important for prevention programs like Fast Track, when failing to screen in a child who develops later antisocial behavior has large costs to society because of that individual's future criminal behavior. The trade-off between sensitivity and specificity across different cut points of a test can be graphed onto a curve known as the ROC (receiver operating characteristic) of a test (e.g., Black, Panzer, Mayewski, & Griner, 1991; McFall & Treat, 1999). ROC curves can be helpful in determining optimal cut points or, if different screening systems are being considered, multiple curves can compare the effectiveness of various systems.

Not all children who exhibit early aggression move on to develop later CD or antisocial behavior (Cicchetti & Richters, 1993; Dodge, 1993), resulting in false positives for screening. Some children may screen in for short-term problems due to family stressors or other circumstances, who recover without intervention as their situations improve. For others, protective factors such as a positive role model and mentor or academic success may help them shift away from a trajectory of developmental risk. In addition, some children become antisocial in later life without displaying early conduct problems (false negatives, often called "late starters").

In reality, the severity of early aggression is a matter of degree, but screening procedures call for a categorical outcome, thus necessitating decisions about cut points to define high-risk status. The cut point used to determine risk status and the base rates of the outcome both affect the accuracy of a screening system. Bennett and colleagues (1999; Bennett & Offord, 2001) have set criteria of at least 50% sensitivity and 50% PPV as minimally adequate to justify screening for an indicated prevention program. These screening values require at least 50% of children who are identified with high levels of early aggression to actually develop later antisocial behavior or CD (PPV), and they require at least 50% of the children who develop later antisocial behavior or CD to be in the screened-in high-risk group (sensitivity). Using the Fast Track data, we conducted a series of studies to evaluate how well our screening system did in reaching these goals, and we also explored the utility of other screening decisions we could have made by studying the normative sample.

In general, we found that the Fast Track multiple gating procedure was effective in predicting to externalizing behavior problems reported by teachers and parents at the end of first grade (Lochman & CPPRG, 1995) and at the end of elementary school (fourth and fifth grades) (Hill et al., 2004). The screening system was also effective in predicting to self-reported delinquency and disruptive behavior diagnoses at the end of elementary school (Hill et al., 2004), and to children's mental health service use and special education involvement in sixth grade (Jones, Dodge, Foster, Nix, & CPPRG, 2002). For example, using the combined parent–teacher ratings of aggression assessed at end of kindergarten to predict poor outcomes at the end of first grade, we found that 70% of the high-risk group had problematic outcomes, whereas 30% had adequate outcomes (Lochman & CPPRG, 1995). This level of prediction of negative outcomes was 3.5 times higher than the rate of problem outcomes in the low-risk groups (21%).

In the course of our analyses, we explored a variety of factors that can influence screening, including (1) source of behavioral ratings and whether both teacher and parent reports are necessary; (2) the timing of screening at the beginning of elementary school; (3) sex differences; and (4) optimization of screening components.

## Source of Behavioral Ratings

An important cost consideration is whether to use teacher-only or combined parent–teacher measures for screening. We examined whether the teacher screen and the parent screen obtained during kindergarten could reliably predict an aggregate of teacher- and parent-reported externalizing behavior problems at the entrance to and end of first grade (Lochman & CPPRG, 1995). Our findings pointed to the usefulness and the relative validity of a two-step multiple-gating screening for kindergarten-age children (i.e., use of both teacher and parent screens) who are at risk for subsequent externalizing problems during the following school year. We should also note that we compared the formal two-gate screening approach with the sum screening approach actually used in Fast Track. In the sum screening approach, the teacher screen and parent screen scores were standardized and summed, creating a sum screen score. The prediction accuracy for the sum screening approach was not significantly different from the two-gate screening approach when examining externalizing problem outcomes at entry to and at the end of first grade.

The parent screen added significant predictive value to the effectiveness of the teacher screen in the regression analyses predicting to first-grade problem behavior; the parent screen accounted for about half as much variance as the teacher screen in predicting to outcomes (Lochman & CPPRG, 1995). Overall, the teacher screen had better sensitivity than did the parent screen (.71 and .51, respectively), indicating that the teacher screen was better at identifying a high percentage of the children who actually had negative outcomes. However, the parent screen had a lower false positive rate (30% vs. 46%), indicating that it was better at excluding ultimately nonproblematic children in those screened as at risk. These analyses indicated the relative advantages of including both teacher and parent reports when predicting to proximal outcomes 1 year later.

However, we have found that the parent screen showed less added value in predicting to later timepoints. Jones and colleagues (2002) examined how the teacher and parent components of the kindergarten screening predicted sixth-grade mental health service use and special education classification. They demonstrated that costly social service utilization (mental health, special education, and juvenile justice involvement) through early adolescence was predicted to a considerable degree by the kindergarten teacher screen. Although the parent screen also showed some predictive power, the high-risk classification derived solely from teacher ratings was as effective in predicting later service use as classification based on both teacher and parent reports. Predictive accuracy was similar across groups defined by child sex and race, and by the four Fast Track sites.

Another study examined how parent and teacher screening predicted fourth- and fifth-grade externalizing behavior (aggregated parent and teacher reports), self-reported delinquency, and disruptive behavior diagnoses using the Diagnostic Interview Schedule for Children (DISC; Hill et al., 2004). For these outcomes, models that included both teacher and parent ratings (first grade only, or a combination of kindergarten plus first grade) had the highest prediction to later combined teacher-plus-parent ratings of externalizing problems and were statistically superior to teacher-only screening models. However, consistent with the findings of Jones and colleagues (2002), teacher-only screening models had high predictive value both for parent–teacher reported externalizing behavior problems and for self-reported delinquency outcomes.

### Timing of Screening at the Beginning of Elementary School

The 2004 study by Hill and colleagues also compared the effectiveness of screening in kindergarten versus first grade. A cross-year screen that included both teacher and parent ratings in both the kindergarten and first-grade years was the most effective predictor of later problem behaviors. However, this full model was not significantly more effective than just relying on teacher and parents in first grade alone. First-grade screening data were notably more accurate than were kindergarten screens in effectively predicting later externalizing behavior problems and delinquency outcomes in fourth and fifth grades. This finding is consistent with results reported by Bennett and Offord (2001), who found higher screening accuracy for their 8- and 9-year-old cohort than for their 5- and 6-year-old cohort. Although intervention strategies have focused on identifying at-risk children as early as possible, first grade may be a better point for screening than kindergarten simply because the task demands of first grade resemble later school experience more closely. In addition to changing situational demands, children's maturing self-regulatory abilities may contribute to the greater predictive power of first-grade predictors.

### Sex Differences

As expected, the various antisocial outcomes examined in Fast Track are between two to four times more prevalent among boys than girls (Hill et al., 2004). For example, for parent and teacher ratings of antisocial outcomes, the prevalence for boys was 2.3 times the rate for girls (16% vs. 7%). For diagnosed externalizing disorders, the rate was almost 3 times higher for boys than for girls (26% vs. 9%); and for self-reported delinquency, the rate was 4 times higher for boys than girls (37% vs. 9%). Correspondingly, the prediction of later antisocial outcomes in Fast Track is more accurate for boys, who are more likely to develop antisocial outcomes. This may be because girls' externalizing behaviors, which tend to be less severe, are correspondingly less stable. Thus, girls "fall out" of a high-risk category at a greater frequency and are more easily misclassified.

Interestingly, the use of a teacher screen that included broader measures of children's early behavioral risk (hyperactive–impulsive and prosocial behaviors, in addition to aggressive behaviors) was more effective than teacher-rated aggression alone in predicting school maladjustment among girls in the Fast Track sample (Flanagan, Bierman, Kam, & CPPRG, 2003). This finding is consistent with research suggesting that at-risk girls may be underdetected when overt aggressive behaviors are used as the primary criteria for risk (Hill et al., 2004; Zoccolillo, Tremblay, & Vitaro, 1996), and that the use of broader measures of early risk may be especially important for girls. The possibility that different kinds of early conduct problems are more predictive for boys and girls is also supported by another Fast Track study. When specific items from the TOCA-R kindergarten teacher screen were examined (Wu et al., 2012), overt behaviors such as "harms others," "fights," and "breaks things" were more predictive for boys, whereas nonphysical behaviors such as "takes property," "stubborn," and "yells at others" were more predictive for girls. Despite these sex differences, however, sex did not appear to affect the predictive utility of the TOCA-R in longitudinal item response theory (IRT) analyses (Racz et al., 2013). These findings do suggest, though, that caution should be used in solely applying the TOCA-R teacher screen with girls.

## Optimization of Screening Components

Despite the findings that support the value of the two-gate screening system used in Fast Track, we were also interested in how to further optimize screening. One way that this could be done would be to focus on screening in first grade rather than kindergarten. Another focus for optimization might be to evaluate the item characteristics of the screening instruments. In the IRT analyses of the TOCA-R teacher screen noted above, we found that the TOCA-R did function fairly well as a measure of conduct problems, but that the original scaling was not ideal (Wu et al., 2012). It could be that teachers found it hard to distinguish between categorical ratings of "often" and "very often," or that fewer categories were required at the severe end ("often" and "very often") to distinguish which children were more or less severe on the latent trait. The analyses indicated that these two categories of "often" and "very often" could be collapsed to create stronger predictions in the IRT analyses.

In a related study, we examined whether the IRT scores for each item would predict broader school behavior outcomes (behavior problems, social competence, academic and disciplinary records), externalizing diagnosis outcomes (ADHD, ODD, CD), and substance use outcomes at the three time points of late childhood, middle adolescence, and late adolescence (Racz et al., 2013). The IRT scores were compared to the typical TOCA-R sum score we had used in the actual Fast Track screening. Higher IRT TOCA-R kindergarten scores consistently predicted more behavior problems at school, lower social skills, and poorer school adjustment reported by multiple informants (teacher, parent, and child) at the end of elementary, middle, and high school. The IRT TOCA-R scores were also related, although somewhat more inconsistently, to the odds of an ADHD diagnosis in ninth grade, as well as ADHD symptoms in sixth and ninth grades, but not to an ODD diagnosis or symptoms or any substance use outcomes. Importantly, when compared to the IRT TOCA-R scores, the screening sum scores demonstrated similar predictive validity to the study outcomes, in spite of the superior psychometric properties of the IRT scores. These findings suggest that in applied settings, such as schools or community mental health centers, or when a quick screening of behavior problems is needed, the calculation of a sum score on the TOCA-R may be sufficient to determine which children are at risk for later problems. However, for statistical analyses using the TOCA-R, IRT scores may be more appropriate given their advantageous distributional properties (Embretson & Reise, 2000).

## LONG-TERM ACCURACY OF FAST TRACK SCREENING

We conducted additional studies to evaluate the long-term accuracy of Fast Track screening in terms of its prediction of adolescent psychopathology (diagnoses of CD) and adult criminal activity. Focusing first on youths' externalizing disorder diagnoses throughout high school (CPPRG, 2011), the combined teacher–parent screen score proved to be a strong predictor. Among children who had the highest scores on this screen score (top 3 percentile), 82% were diagnosed with an externalizing psychiatric disorder, compared with just 32% for the rest of the sample. This top 3% group was also substantially higher in risk than the group between the 90th and 97th percentile (58% prevalence) and the group between the 80th and 90th percentile (50% prevalence). In addition, the Fast Track screen yielded relatively few (only 18%) false negative predictions for later externalizing psychiatric disorder.

Most recently, we have examined the degree to which the Fast Track screen effectively predicted criminal convictions 20 years after initial screening at age 25 (Kassing, Godwin, Lochman, Coie, & CPPRG, 2019). We found that, in our normative sample drawn from high-risk schools, the rate of adult criminal convictions by age 25 was 39.8%—considerably higher than the 20% we anticipated (Hill et al., 2004). Using the 39.8% base rate for analyses, all combinations of the parent and teacher screen scores across the kindergarten and first-grade years met the PPV and sensitivity cutoffs for a well-performing screening tool, as defined in the Hill et al. study. Using the combination of teacher-only kindergarten and first-grade screen scores yielded the best results, but the actual kindergarten-only Fast Track screen score that combined teacher and parent kindergarten screen scores also performed well. Given the possible lower intervention efficacy that would have resulted from waiting a year before beginning intervention, our decision to identify high-risk children during kindergarten seems well grounded in long-term findings. The Fast Track screen was similarly effective in predicting adult arrests in official records and substance use problems as reported by participants or their peers, but less effective at predicting participant-reported psychiatric disorders. Thus, the screen performed best at predicting one of the major outcomes that Fast Track was designed to prevent (i.e., adult arrests), but not ODD or CD outcomes.

When we examined the accuracy of screening within each site separately, Fast Track screening was most effective in Durham and Nashville, where the base rates for criminal conviction were relatively high (48.4% and 47.9%, respectively). In contrast, the base rates in Pennsylvania and Seattle were considerably lower (30.4% and 27.3%, respectively), and the screen scores did not perform as well. However, even in these sites, the use of teacher plus parent ratings in both kindergarten and first grade produced adequate screening; in the sites with higher baselines, a simple screening by a kindergarten teacher would have been sufficient. Prediction models also worked best for males, who had higher base rates of criminal conviction than females.

## SUMMARY

When Fast Track was designed in 1990, we used the best available evidence to develop a screening system that could accurately detect which children were at highest risk for antisocial and criminal outcomes so that we could deliver intensive prevention programming to that group. Twenty-nine years later, a set of predictive studies suggests that the brief teacher and parent screens that were used were effective at identifying youth at high risk, with reasonably low false positive and false negative rates. Thus, with the cooperation of the local school districts in each of the communities, we were able to construct a valid sample of children showing high aggression at school entrance; furthermore, our randomization by school was effective in creating comparable intervention and control groups. In addition, these high-risk children were shown to have later pathways with substantial difficulties as they matured during elementary, middle, and high school.

Screening items that focused on child aggressive behaviors proved sufficient to identify families who also struggled with several other risk factors linked with antisocial developmental risks. These included factors such as low levels of education, financial stress, caregiver depression, unsafe neighborhoods, low levels of social support, single-parent status, and a reliance on harsh discipline practices. It was not necessary to include these risk factors in the screening process, likely because their influence on child development was already reflected in the children's aggression levels at kindergarten entry. Conversely, children who were not exhibiting aggression by then were not likely to respond to the family stressors with aggression in later years (although they might be at risk for other difficulties). The findings reported in this chapter validate the Fast Track screening system, and also reflect the stability and negative predictability of early aggression, especially for children growing up in low-income communities. Without intervention, many of these children grew up to exhibit serious antisocial and criminal behavior.

## FAST TRACK CASE STUDIES

Throughout our work in Fast Track, we have focused on how effective the intervention was with those high-risk youth who participated in the intervention, in comparison to those high-risk youth who did not participate. These youth had kindergarten risk scores that were among the top 20% of all youth assessed. However, as we delivered the intervention, we were constantly aware of the variation within the intervention sample in how youth and parents engaged with Fast Track services; in contextual influences, such as financial, legal, and mental health stressors; and in youth and parent proximal outcomes. Thus, to provide some context for understanding the *between-group* effects of the intervention, which is the main focus of this book, we offer two case stories to illustrate the diversity *within* the intervention sample. These are composite case studies based upon several youth with names and some details altered to preserve participant confidentiality. After introducing each case study here, we share brief descriptions of each youth's and parent's engagement with Fast Track and their proximal outcomes in the forthcoming chapters on implementation and outcomes.

### Jeremiah and Grace Locke*

Jeremiah Locke was an active young black boy who was headstrong and often defiant. In kindergarten, he already showed high levels of aggressive behavior and attention problems in both school and home settings, typical of children whom Fast Track wanted to target. During a home observation, although Jeremiah showed a great deal of warmth toward his mother Grace, she only reciprocated occasionally, giving him limited attention. Grace felt that she was a capable and competent single parent, but found parenting Jeremiah both difficult and anxiety producing. During the summer before Fast Track started, Grace noted that Jeremiah did not comply with her requests, would yell at her, and, at times, was physically aggressive toward her. Along with the stress of disciplining Jeremiah, Grace was coping with a limited income and corresponding financial challenges, as well as a recent move to a dangerous neighborhood rife with substance abuse and drug dealing. In school, Jeremiah was reading at the same level as his peers, but was struggling with basic math concepts. His kindergarten teacher reported that Jeremiah was more aggressive than other children and that he fought, yelled at, and physically hurt his peers.

### Cindy and Susan Steele

Cindy Steele's screen score put her near the top among the girls identified for the Fast Track high-risk sample. Her kindergarten teacher described her as a friendly but very stubborn girl who often broke rules, was disobedient, and teased her peers. Despite attending Head Start, Cindy was struggling with math and reading. In addition to problems with aggression, Cindy had significant attention problems and was also an emotional child, expressing many worries and sad feelings. At home, Cindy shared a physically affectionate relationship with her mother, Susan, but they also fought frequently. Cindy often ignored her mother's requests and was physically aggressive toward her. In turn, Susan found herself yelling at Cindy, threatening punishment, and spanking her on a daily basis. In general,

---

* Names of youth and parents and other potentially identifying information have been changed to protect confidentiality.

Susan felt insecure about her parenting skills, and overwhelmed by the challenges of parenting three children under the age of 6 (Cindy and her two younger sisters). Susan and her partner, Al (who was not Cindy's biological father), worked full time, but still struggled with major financial problems. Susan felt isolated and dissatisfied with her neighborhood. She had little contact with her neighbors or family and wished for more social contact and support.

In the next chapter, we describe the Fast Track preventive intervention, and how it was organized to address the multiple needs evident in this group of high-risk children and their families.

# Chapter 4

# The Fast Track Intervention in the Elementary School Years

This chapter describes the elementary intervention (grades 1–5), when children were (on average) 6–11 years old. Fast Track also included intervention activities that extended from the transition into middle school through the transition into high school (i.e., grades 6–10); these adolescent intervention activities are described in Chapter 6. The elementary intervention included a universal intervention delivered at the classroom level, which served all children in participating schools, along with additional components that were delivered to children identified as high-risk aggressive and their families. Some of the intervention components for high-risk children and families were delivered in a standard fashion, with all participants receiving the same amount and type of intervention, whereas other components were delivered in an adaptive, tailored fashion, with the type or amount of intervention adjusted to child and/or family need based on embedded assessments. The content and delivery of these various intervention components changed over time, to provide supports adjusted for developmental needs and opportunities.

In this chapter, we first describe each of the intervention components. Second, we describe the timing of intervention delivery and the staffing arrangements. Third, we provide implementation data, including amount and quality of implementation and predictors of patterns of child and family engagement in intervention, along with data on the accuracy and impact of tailoring some intervention components. Finally, we provide a summary of lessons learned regarding the design of multicomponent and tailored interventions, and the recruitment and maintenance of engagement among youth, families, and schools.

## COMPONENTS OF THE FAST TRACK ELEMENTARY
## SCHOOL INTERVENTION

The Fast Track intervention design was based on the developmental model of early-starting conduct problems described in Chapter 2 (see also CPPRG, 1992). Accordingly, Fast Track targeted the primary child risk factors for CD evident at school entry, promoting social-emotional competencies to address deficits in self-control, emotion dysregulation, poor peer relations, and weak academic skills. In the later elementary years, an additional goal was the promotion of resilience, feelings of self-efficacy, and a positive racial/ethnic identity for black youth. Fast Track was also designed to improve supports for positive child development in the home context by increasing positive parenting practices, decreasing parent–child conflict and harsh punishment, and improving the quality of the parent–child relationship. In addition, Fast Track sought to improve the classroom atmosphere, reducing classroom disruptiveness, and enhancing the teacher's capacity to provide positive supports to all students in the classroom. A final goal was to improve the quality of teacher–parent communications and increase consistent support for positive child development across the home and school settings. To address these goals, Fast Track combined a number of different intervention approaches that had shown promise in prior, short-term intervention studies.

### Classroom-Level Intervention: The PATHS Curriculum

At the universal level of prevention, teachers taught a grade-level version of the PATHS curriculum (Greenberg, Kusché, & CPPRG, 2011; Kusché et al., 2011), presenting lessons two to three times per week in grades 1–5. The PATHS curriculum is a social-emotional learning (SEL) intervention that targets the domains of prosocial skills (helping, sharing, cooperating), self-control, emotional awareness and understanding, and social problem solving to increase social and emotional competence. In the early school years, targeted skills were designed to enhance adaptation to the rules and routines of school and to foster the development of positive peer relations. In later years, more advanced topics included decision-making skills, study skills, goal setting, character development, coping with peer pressure, and problem-solving skills.

Fast Track included a universal SEL intervention for several reasons. First, providing all children with supports that promote prosocial skills and peaceful conflict resolution should foster a positive classroom atmosphere that supports positive interpersonal relations for all students and reduces peer contagion supporting aggression (Greenberg et al., 2003). In addition, providing teachers with professional development supports that allow them to better manage the classroom should also promote aggression control (Hawkins, Catalano, Kosterman, Abbott, & Hill, 1999; Walker, Colvin, & Ramsey, 1996). By synchronizing universal with indicated interventions for high-risk children, teachers are positioned to support the generalization of the social and self-control skills children are learning in the indicated interventions into the classroom setting. Reciprocally, providing high-risk aggressive children in the classroom with coordinated intensive skill training should reduce their classroom disruptiveness, making both them and their classmates more receptive to the classroom-level programming.

Classroom teachers attended annual 2-day workshops to train them to deliver the PATHS curriculum and received regular consultation from Fast Track staff (described in more detail below) to help them generalize PATHS teaching strategies throughout the day. It was anticipated that the high-risk aggressive children served by Fast Track would benefit from the social-cognitive skills taught in class as well as from the additional positive management support provided by classroom teachers and the improved peer culture in the classroom.

## Friendship Groups for Social Skill Training

High-risk aggressive children were invited to attend Friendship Groups held during an extracurricular enrichment program (explained below), designed to work in parallel with the PATHS curriculum and provide more intensive skill training. Friendship Groups targeted children's prosocial skills, emotional expression and emotional understanding, accurate awareness of others' intentions, anger control, emotional regulation, and social problem-solving skills. Based on prior intervention research, it was anticipated that these groups would address deficits in positive social interaction skills and promote improvements in the areas of social-cognitive distortions and deficiencies that are common among aggressive children (Bierman, 2004; Coie & Koeppl, 1990; Lochman, Coie, Underwood, & Terry, 1993).

Coaching methods (i.e., direct instruction, modeling, behavioral rehearsal, and multiple opportunities to practice skills with performance feedback) were used to build skills (Bierman & Powers, 2009). Role playing and videotaping reinforced the use of more competent social problem-solving skills, and positive behavior management strategies reinforced positive behavioral goals and effective self-regulation (see also Bierman, 2004). Additional details about Friendship Groups are provided in Bierman, Greenberg, and CPPRG (1996), and the Friendship Group manual is now published and available (Bierman, Greenberg, et al., 2017).

### Peer Pairing

The Friendship Group sessions were held outside of the school day. For this reason, an additional intervention component was designed to promote the generalization of new social skills to the school setting and to help children build more positive relationships with classroom peers. Prior research suggested that including classmates in social skill training sessions and facilitating engagement in cooperative activities could promote positive changes in classmate behavior and attitudes toward rejected children (Bierman, 1986; Bierman & Furman, 1984). The peer-pairing component of Fast Track used this strategy. High-risk aggressive children were provided with a supervised half-hour play session with classroom peers each week, scheduled at a time that was convenient for the teacher, and focused on practicing skills introduced in Friendship Group sessions. Classmate partners were selected based on their positive classroom behavior and rotated over the course of the year. In addition to providing high-risk children with social skill practice, a key goal was to expose multiple classmates to the improved behavior and prosocial skills of the high-risk aggressive children during cooperative activities, which has been associated with improved peer reputations and peer status (Bierman & Furman, 1984). In first grade, peer pairing was offered to all high-risk aggressive children. In second grade, it was offered to the subset of children who continued to experience peer rejection or exhibit high rates of aggression toward peers at assessments conducted at the end of first grade, based on peer sociometric nominations and teacher ratings. In the later elementary years (grades 3–5) peer support was offered to children with ongoing social needs through a weekly "social club" or "lunch club" offered after school or during an indoor recess period.

### PARENT GROUPS AND PARENT–CHILD SHARING SESSIONS

Parent Groups were also included as a core component of Fast Track, based on prior evidence demonstrating the efficacy of positive behavior management training in clinic settings for parents of children with early oppositional or conduct disorders (e.g., McMahon & Frick, 2019). Although individual parent management training programs vary considerably in the specific intervention procedures and activities they use, all share a common focus on enhancing parent skills at providing clear expectations and directions to their children, positively reinforcing positive child behavior with specific praise and other rewards, and using nonpunitive discipline strategies to correct misbehaviors (e.g., time out, response cost, privilege removal, contingency contract).

Primarily, parent management training programs were developed to serve families attending clinics (or referred to clinics) who were experiencing significant difficulties managing their children's behavior. A key difference in designing Fast Track was that parents did not initiate help seeking, but rather were identified for support based upon the child behavior screening. A second difference was that, in addition to addressing behavior management issues, Fast Track sought to address other key developmental issues faced by children who enter school with high rates of aggression. These included parental support in meeting the learning challenges of early elementary school (grades 1 and 2), including learning to read, follow rules, get along with others, feel good about themselves, and become self-regulated.

Accordingly, the Fast Track Parent Groups focused on improving positive parent–child interactions, reducing harsh and punitive discipline, and increasing consistent limit setting by teaching effective communication and positive discipline skills (including praise and ignoring, clear instructions and rules, and time out) based on previously validated evidence-based programs (Forehand & McMahon, 1981; Webster-Stratton, 1984). Fast Track Parent Groups also sought to promote the development of positive family–school relationships, enhance parent self-control and feelings of parental self-efficacy, foster developmentally appropriate expectations, and foster parents' abilities to support child engagement and adjustment at school. Consistent with the screening and recruitment strategy used in Fast Track, initial Parent Group sessions focused on helping children get off to a good start in school. Behavior management topics were placed later in the year. Across years, topics shifted to include developmentally relevant parenting challenges. For example, there was a gradual shift from parent-initiated behavior management strategies in the early elementary school years to an increasing focus in grades 4 and 5 on parent–child communication and problem-solving strategies and parental monitoring to address emergent issues such as deviant peers, substance use, and sexuality. Sessions incorporated discussions, video examples, and role-play exercises to teach new strategies and present alternative means of handling common child-rearing challenges. Additional details about Parent Groups are provided in McMahon, Slough, and CPPRG (1996), and the Parent Group manual is in preparation for publication (McMahon et al., 2019).

## Parent–Child Sharing

During the initial years of the intervention, Fast Track Parent Group sessions were followed by Parent–Child Sharing sessions. Parent–Child Sharing sessions had two goals: (1) to foster positive parent–child relationships through the promotion of positive, cooperative parent–child interactions; and (2) to provide parents with an opportunity to practice the skills introduced in Parent Groups with staff guidance. The skill topics addressed in the parent and child groups followed a developmental sequence, with an increasing emphasis over time on communication skills, homework study skills, goal setting, and negotiating parent–child conflicts.

Typically, Parent–Child Sharing sessions started with a story chosen to highlight a theme introduced by PATHS, Friendship Groups, or Parent Groups, and served to promote parent–child reading and set the stage for parent–child interaction activities that followed the stories. After the story, parents and children participated in guided cooperative activities, games, or crafts. These activities were designed to reinforce skills introduced in PATHS or Friendship Groups, such as identifying and expressing emotions, and using social problem-solving skills. The activities were also structured to allow parents to practice skills introduced in the Parent Group such as providing positive child-oriented attention, stating positive expectations, and setting effective limits. Each session ended with a complimenting exercise adapted from PATHS, in which each parent complimented his or her child on an aspect of the child's behavior, effort, or accomplishment, and each child complimented her or his parent, focusing on a parent behavior, effort, or accomplishment during the past week.

## Home Visiting

Fast Track home visits had several goals. First, home visits provided intervention staff with an opportunity to meet other family members, better understand each family's system and family situation, and build a strong, individual working alliance with each primary caregiver. Second, home visits provided an opportunity to review the parenting skills with each family by discussing the relevance and strategies for use in that particular family context. In addition, barriers to effective parenting were addressed, including contextual influences or personal situations that made it challenging for the parent(s) to utilize effective parenting strategies. Third, home visits focused on strengthening parent–school engagement, as intervention staff served as a communication liaison between home and school, and by helping parents support child schooling at home (e.g., encouraging parent–child reading at home, support for homework completion). Finally, home visits provided opportunities to address pressing family issues via referral to other community supports and problem-solving discussions. In this area, following the model developed by Wasik and colleagues (Wasik, Bryant, & Lyons, 1990), Fast Track focused on promoting parent problem solving, coping, and goal setting in order to deal with the multiple stressful events the families often faced (e.g., marital conflict, substance abuse, social isolation, and housing and employment issues). The goal of this problem-solving approach was to promote parent feelings of efficacy and self-sufficiency in managing family stressors and moving forward in areas of family and parenting goals.

As noted, during the child's first-grade year, attempts were made to visit all families every other week and to contact families weekly by phone. In subsequent years, the Family Coordinators (FCs) who conducted Parent Groups and home visits completed a brief, six-item form to evaluate family strengths and risks three times each year (September, January, May). The score on this assessment, along with FC and supervisor discussion, was used to set the recommended level of family home visiting for the subsequent 4 months. Home visiting could be recommended at varying levels of intensity—weekly, biweekly, or monthly.

## Academic Tutoring

Fast Track also included an academic tutoring program, based on prior evidence that tutoring could reduce the cognitive delays of early-starting aggressive children and improve their school adjustment in elementary school (Coie & Krehbiel, 1984). Young children growing up in disadvantaged circumstances who exhibit elevated aggressive-disruptive behavior often also show delays in cognitive functioning that reduce school readiness, including low reading readiness, elevated attention problems, and low cognitive ability (Hinshaw, 1992; Moffitt, 1993). Accordingly, all high-risk children received tutoring in reading skills during first grade, using an evidence-based phonics approach—the Wallach reading tutoring program (Wallach & Wallach, 1976). This highly structured one-on-one tutoring program was designed for use by paraprofessionals to serve low-readiness children from disadvantaged backgrounds, and emphasized a phonics-based, mastery-oriented approach to the development of initial reading skills.

All high-risk children received three tutoring sessions per week in first grade. In the subsequent years after children had completed the

Wallach reading program, tutoring was provided to children who were struggling academically, performing in the bottom third of the class based on teacher report. Once children had mastered the Wallach program, tutoring focused increasingly on homework completion and other learning activities recommended by the classroom teacher. In the later elementary years (grades 3–5), tutoring was commonly provided outside of the regular school day, during a homework club held after school twice per week. These sessions typically involved a snack, time spent with tutors focused on homework completion and studying, and then group games.

## Mentoring

Finally, Fast Track included a mentoring program in the later elementary school years (i.e., grades 4 and 5). The goal was to provide a same-sex, same-race community volunteer mentor for children who lacked an appropriate same-sex, same-race adult role model in their life. The general goal was to promote a positive racial/ethnic identity, a strong sense of efficacy, and to foster the development of personal goals and aspirations for the future, as well as to strengthen social support in the child's community. This was a component of Fast Track that proved quite difficult to implement, due to the difficulty involved in finding a sufficient number of volunteer mentors. In the later years of the program, some mentors were paid. Due to the difficulty in finding mentors, rates of mentoring declined in a linear fashion over time, with most children who qualified for mentoring in cohort 1 but very few children who qualified for mentoring in cohort 3 receiving mentoring. Hence, mentoring is not considered a core component of the Fast Track program.

Fast Track intervention services were intensive as children entered elementary school (grades 1 and 2), designed to reduce skill deficits evident at school entry in kindergarten and build the child and family competencies needed for successful school adjustment. Standard intervention services then decreased to a maintenance schedule during the later elementary years (grades 3–5), with tailored individualized services offered at more intensive levels based on ongoing assessments of child and family need. Figure 4.1 illustrates the core components that all Fast Track children and families were offered in the elementary schools. As noted above, mentoring was initiated for some children in the later elementary years (grade 4), corresponding to the developmental increase in the influence of the self-system on behavioral control and mental health.

As noted earlier, PATHS was taught by classroom teachers in intervention schools from grades 1–5 (Greenberg et al., 2011). Fast Track staff also met with teachers individually, to provide consultation regarding

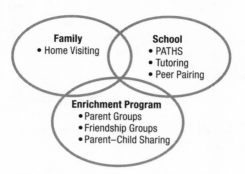

**FIGURE 4.1.** Core components of the Fast Track elementary school intervention.

the implementation of the PATHS curriculum and offer support in the design of effective classroom behavior management programs for high-risk aggressive children.

## Enrichment Sessions

Families with identified high-risk aggressive children were invited to attend weekly, 2-hour extracurricular enrichment sessions that were held regularly at local schools in the late afternoon, evening, or on Saturday. These enrichment sessions included separate group meetings for parents (Parent Groups) and children (Friendship Groups), as well as the Parent–Child Sharing session. In first grade, Parent and Friendship Groups were 60 minutes long, followed by a tutoring session that parents observed. In later years, Parent and Friendship Groups were 90 minutes long. Across these years, the last 30 minutes of each session brought parents and children together for joint activities (Parent–Child Sharing). Extracurricular enrichment sessions were held weekly (22 sessions) in grade 1, biweekly (14 sessions) in grade 2, and monthly (8 sessions) each year in grades 3–5.

Additional tailored indicated interventions were delivered in a standard fashion the first year of intervention. In subsequent years, criterion-referenced assessments were used to adjust the dosage of these three indicated components to match the level of functioning of each family and child. As noted above, these included peer-pairing sessions held at school, designed to facilitate the generalization of social skills and help children build friendships within the school setting, and academic tutoring sessions focused on promoting reading readiness and basic literacy skills. All families received regular home visits to help parents apply the skills presented in the group setting, but after first grade, the frequency varied depending upon family need. The timing and number of sessions offered across these components is summarized in Table 4.1.

### Intervention Staffing

The two core Fast Track intervention staff positions were Educational Coordinators (ECs) and Family Coordinators (FCs). In addition, paraprofessional staff were hired to assist ECs with the school-based intervention components, and both Friendship Groups and Parent Groups had group coleaders.

The ECs at each site were experienced classroom teachers who had

**TABLE 4.1. Fast Track Core Components Delivery Schedule**

| Components | Grade 1 | Grade 2 | Grade 3 | Grade 4 | Grade 5 |
|---|---|---|---|---|---|
| | | | Universal components | | |
| PATHS curriculum | 2×/week (52 sessions) | 2×/week (46 sessions) | 2×/week (48 sessions) | 2×/week (35 sessions) | 2×/week (35 sessions) |
| | | | Indicated components | | |
| Friendship Group | Weekly | Biweekly | Monthly | Monthly | Monthly |
| Parent Group | Weekly | Biweekly | Monthly | Monthly | Monthly |
| Parent–Child Sharing | Weekly (22 sessions) | Biweekly (14 sessions) | Monthly (8 sessions) | Monthly (8 sessions) | Monthly (8 sessions) |
| Mentoring | | | | Weekly (36 sessions) | Weekly (36 sessions) |
| | | | Tailored components | | |
| Home visits | Biweekly (11 sessions) | Varied (9–36 sessions) | Varied (9–36 sessions) | Varied (9–36 sessions) | Varied (9–36 sessions) |
| Peer pairing/ social club | Weekly (22 sessions) | Yes/No (0–14 sessions) | Yes/No (0–14 sessions) | Yes/No (0–14 sessions) | Yes/No (0–14 sessions) |
| Academic tutoring | 3×/week (60 sessions) | Yes/No (0–60 sessions) | Yes/No (0–60 sessions) | Yes/No (0–60 sessions) | Yes/No (0–60 sessions) |

*Note.* Varied levels of home visits included weekly, biweekly, or monthly, based on assessments of family need. Numbers in parentheses represent planned sessions.

expertise working with behaviorally challenging children. ECs delivered the social skill training (Friendship Groups) to target children, supervised paraprofessionals in the implementation of the tutoring and peer-pairing programs, and consulted with classroom teachers on PATHS implementation and classroom management issues. In their role as teacher consultants, ECs made weekly visits to each classroom and met with teachers each month either individually or in small groups. ECs reviewed the implementation of PATHS with teachers, modeled classroom lessons, and discussed classroom management challenges, offering support in planning and implementing positive behavior management programs. ECs received 3 days of cross-site training each year, and followed detailed manuals describing the assessment and intervention protocols for each of the key program components. They were supervised in weekly meetings at each site; supervisors participated in weekly cross-site phone calls with the particular principal investigators who oversaw the key program components.

The FCs at each site were women with advanced degrees and/or many years of experience working in human services. Women were hired for this role because many of the primary caregivers were single mothers who we felt would feel most comfortable with another woman visiting them in their homes. To strengthen the likelihood that staff could develop positive working relationships with high-risk families, an attempt was made to recruit professional staff with similar cultural and ethnic backgrounds as the families (Orrell-Valente, Pinderhughes, Valente, Laird, & CPPRG, 1999). FCs led the Parent Groups and Parent–Child Sharing sessions, and conducted home visits with parents. FCs from all sites met for joint training during a 3-day cross-site training workshop held each year during the elementary school intervention. FCs within each site also participated in ongoing group and individual supervision, conducted weekly with an on-site supervisor. Supervisors participated in weekly cross-site phone calls with the particular principal investigators who oversaw the key program components. They followed a detailed manual for each Parent Group and Parent–Child Sharing session, so content was always similar across Parent Groups. They also followed guidelines in the conduct of their home visits, although these visits were individualized by design to allow FCs to tailor the content to support the parent's capacity to use the parenting skills effectively in their personal situation. ECs and FCs worked in pairs, serving an average of 15–18 families.

## Paraprofessional Staff and Group Coleaders

Paraprofessional staff were recruited from each community to provide in-school peer-pairing and tutoring sessions. School personnel often assisted in the recruitment of these individuals. Many of them were already working with children in the school setting, and had prior experience working in schools. In some cases, retired teachers served in this role; in other cases, paraprofessionals filled this role. Tutors received 40 hours of training and ongoing supervision. Group coleaders who helped manage the Friendship Group and Parent Group sessions were typically graduate students or undergraduate students with experience working with children. Some of these individuals were graduate or undergraduate students in training; others were recruited and selected by the ECs and FCs, who trained and supervised them.

### Mentors

Mentors were primarily volunteers recruited from the communities where the high-risk aggressive children lived. A Mentor Coordinator at each site was responsible for recruiting, training, and supervising the volunteer mentors. In some cases, particularly the rural site where children lived in isolated areas and small towns that did not have the population density to support the recruitment of sufficient numbers of mentors, mentors also included hired staff (typically college students) who traveled to the rural communities to provide mentoring.

## INTERVENTION IMPLEMENTATION IN THE ELEMENTARY YEARS

The initial challenge was to engage families in the intervention. As detailed in Chapter 3, all families (intervention and control groups) were recruited in the same way into the Fast Track developmental study. In the fall of first grade, recruited parents of children attending schools randomized to the intervention condition were subsequently invited to participate in the full intervention. In other words, when families agreed to participate in the developmental study, they did not know that an intervention would be offered. Hence, Fast Track intervention staff had the task of engaging children and families into the various intervention components. In the following sections, we first describe patterns of participation in the school-based intervention components (PATHS, academic tutoring, peer pairing). Then, we describe patterns of participation in the extracurricular intervention components (Parent Group and Parent–Child Sharing, Friendship Group, home visits, mentoring). Finally, we present findings from research conducted to better understand the predictors of participation and the associations with intervention outcomes.

## Implementation of the School-Based Intervention Components

Implementation of the school-based intervention components depended heavily on the cooperation of school personnel, as teachers were responsible for delivery of the PATHS curriculum and facilitating the scheduling of pull-out tutoring and peer-pairing sessions. Over time, child involvement in the school-based intervention activities depended largely on the child's ongoing enrollment in schools where services could be delivered, and on the Fast Track staff's capacity to work effectively with schools to schedule and complete planned sessions. Prior to the initiation of the Fast Track program, meetings were held with school administrators (superintendents, principals, school boards) and with teachers at each elementary school. In general, school personnel were very interested in the program and especially welcomed the parent-focused components (Parent Group and home-visiting services), as these were services that they generally lacked the resources and expertise to offer. Almost all schools contacted about the project wanted to participate. At the same time, once schools were randomized, some teachers voiced concerns about the time requirements and usefulness of both the PATHS curriculum and the pull-out tutoring and peer-pairing sessions. To promote teacher buy-in, Fast Track emphasized the importance of building strong working alliances between ECs and teachers. All ECs had teaching experience themselves, which gave them some face validity in the school setting. Their schedule included time in each classroom: ECs were encouraged to make weekly visits to classrooms, in order to observe and model PATHS lessons and help teachers problem solve about behavior management issues. During the first year of program implementation at each grade level, ECs also met weekly with teachers individually or in small groups. By building strong working relationships with teachers, taking time to understand their classroom context, and providing them with opportunities to voice their opinions, it was easier for ECs to negotiate implementation challenges, such as time constraints, scheduling of pull-out sessions, and classroom management.

Unfortunately for Fast Track, the Durham City school district underwent a major reorganization after the second year of the trial, merging with the Durham County school district and reassigning children to new schools. This reorganization completely confounded the randomized school assignment to intervention versus control conditions. The implementation of PATHS continued in the Durham schools originally randomized to the intervention; however, we were unable to include the Durham schools in longitudinal analyses of the impact of the universal intervention because of this shift in the school-based samples.

The Fast Track strategies were generally successful in promoting the high-quality implementation of the PATHS curriculum. Across the elementary school years, the mean number of lessons taught ranged from 80% to 92%, with higher average levels at the earlier grade levels. Fidelity was assessed using monthly ratings completed by ECs, who used their direct observations as well as discussions with teachers to rate the quality of curriculum delivery and generalization throughout the day. These fidelity ratings included four aspects of PATHS implementation: (1) quality of teaching of PATHS concepts, (2) modeling of PATHS concepts throughout the day, (3) quality of classroom management (during PATHS lessons), and (4) openness to consultation from the EC. Each dimension was rated on a 4-point scale (from *low skilled* to *highly skilled performance*). Fidelity was relatively constant across grade levels, averaging 3.2 for quality of teaching concepts, 3.0 for modeling of PATHS concepts, 3.1 for classroom management, and 3.0 for openness to consultation (CPPRG, 2010c).

Positive working relationships with teachers also facilitated the scheduling of pull-out sessions for peer pairing and tutoring. All but three children received some tutoring in first grade, with an average of 50 sessions delivered (83% of the planned amount). In the subsequent years, on average, two-thirds of the children in the sample qualified for tutoring each year, and over 80% of those who qualified received tutoring each year. By third grade, most of these sessions were held after school in a "homework club" scheduled twice a week. The major impediment to tutoring was that children moved out of schools where tutoring could be delivered; this number of children who moved increased by about 5% each year. Of those who received tutoring, the average number of sessions was 40 per year during the elementary years. After first grade when all children qualified for peer pairing, it was continued for an additional year for children with significant ongoing peer difficulties. Rates of peer-pairing participation in second grade were equivalent to tutoring participation. Participation rates for tutoring and peer pairing are shown in Table 4.2.

## Implementation of the Extracurricular Intervention Components

Engaging parents and children in the extracurricular components of Fast Track involved additional challenges and efforts that extended well beyond those needed to manage the school-based intervention components. In general, research suggests that it is very difficult to recruit and retain multiproblem families in family-focused interventions (Sanders & Markie-Dadds, 1992). In addition, on average, 30% of the families who

**TABLE 4.2. Participation in Academic Tutoring and Peer Pairing in Grades 2–4**

| Grade level | % recommended for service | | Of those recommended, % sessions attended | | Of those recommended, % attending half or more | |
| --- | --- | --- | --- | --- | --- | --- |
| | Tutoring | Peer pairing | Tutoring | Peer pairing | Tutoring | Peer pairing |
| Grade 2 | 68% | 44% | 66% | 66% | 80% | 81% |
| Grade 3 | 66% | NA | 62% | NA | 72% | NA |
| Grade 4 | 60% | NA | 68% | NA | 83% | NA |
| Grade 5 | 63% | NA | 65% | NA | 75% | NA |

*Note.* Tutoring in grades 2 and 3 was recommended for children who were in the lower third in their class for reading ability. Sixty sessions were recommended per year (two to three times per week).

begin parenting interventions drop out before completing the programs (Forehand, Middlebrook, Rogers, & Steffe, 1983). Given the multiple components and length of the Fast Track program, along with the fact that parents were not necessarily seeking out intervention when they were recruited, we paid particular attention to reducing barriers and increasing motivation to encourage parent engagement. For example, the intervention was described to parents as providing enrichment and support to help their children succeed at school, and all components were explained in terms of their competency-building orientation. Extracurricular program sessions were scheduled to maximize match with parent availability. For parents who were reluctant to attend the Parent Group sessions, FCs were patient and would revisit the issue when parents appeared more open to this service. Transportation and child care for siblings were provided, refreshments were offered, and, in recognition of the time involved for parents and their investment in the professional development training activities, parents were compensated $15 per family per session attended.

In general, these strategies were very successful in engaging parents and encouraging parent attendance at the extracurricular sessions. Only a few families declined to initiate participation in the Parent Groups or Friendship Groups in first grade; 95% of parents and 98% of children attended at least one group session. Of those who participated, 79% of the parents and 90% of the children attended at least half of the sessions. Participation declined slightly over the subsequent years, due primarily to family moves, but remained fairly strong (see Table 4.3 for participation rates). Note that "parent" is used generically here to refer to the

**TABLE 4.3. Participation in Parent Groups and Friendship Groups in Grades 1–5**

| Grade level | % attending any sessions | | % sessions attended | | % attending half or more | |
|---|---|---|---|---|---|---|
| | Parent | Child | Parent | Child | Parent | Child |
| Grade 1 (22 sessions) | 95 | 98 | 70 | 77 | 79 | 90 |
| Grade 2 (14 sessions) | 78 | 85 | 63 | 73 | 75 | 85 |
| Grade 3 (8 sessions) | 72 | 80 | 67 | 77 | 81 | 90 |
| Grade 4 (8 sessions) | 63 | 76 | 67 | 77 | 78 | 87 |
| Grade 5 (8 sessions) | 60 | 74 | 63 | 73 | 75 | 85 |

primary caregivers; all adults who were involved in child rearing were invited to attend these sessions.

Fast Track also included measures reflecting the quality of Parent Group and Friendship Group participation. In Parent Groups, FCs rated the quality of parent participation in both the Parent Groups and Parent–Child Sharing sessions using scales adapted from prior research (Dumas, Nissley-Tsiopinis, & Moreland, 2007; Karver, Handelsman, Fields, & Bickman, 2005) that tapped dimensions such as listening attentively, asking questions when appropriate, being receptive to new ways of interacting with children, and actively contributing to discussions and role plays. Ratings of participation quality were only somewhat correlated with rate of attendance ($r = 0.38$) and they showed considerable variation across individuals, suggesting that it was easier to promote consistent attendance than to promote consistently high-quality participation at Parent Groups (for more detail, see Nix, Bierman, McMahon, & CPPRG, 2009).

The quality of each child's participation in a Friendship Group was also measured. ECs used a 4-point scale to rate in-session interactions, including (1) child positive behaviors (e.g., friendly overtures, helping, sharing, problem solving), (2) child negative behaviors (e.g., disruptive, noncompliant, aggressive), (3) peer encouragement (e.g., positive peer behaviors toward child), and (4) peer escalation of negative behavior (e.g., peer responses reinforcing negative child behavior, including laughing, imitating, or fighting back). EC ratings indicated that 54% of the child participants received high scores for positive in-session behavior (average of 3–4), and 79% received low scores for negative in-session behavior (average of 1–2). At the other end of the spectrum, a small number of children showed poor-quality participation in Friendship Groups, with 5% showing little positive behavior (average of 1–2), and 3% displayed chronic challenging behaviors (average of 3–4). Peer responses were positive and supportive for 75% of the children (average of 3–4), but a few children (5%) regularly received peer responses that reinforced negative behavior in the Friendship Group setting. Positive behavior management strategies received a high level of attention in the Fast Track curriculum, staff training, and supervision process. The positive quality of most children's engagement in Friendship Groups suggests that, with a structured skill-training program and positive behavior management by staff, a therapeutic context was achieved in most groups, even though they were comprised of aggressive children. At the same time, behavior management required extensive efforts in about 20% of the groups, and management strategies were ineffective in 5% of the groups, likely due to the peer deviancy training that can emerge in groups composed solely of aggressive children (Dishion & Tipsord, 2011).

## Home Visit Participation

While parents were scheduled to be visited on a biweekly basis in first grade, starting in second grade, families were recommended for different levels of home visiting. About half of the sample was recommended for biweekly home visiting during the school year (8–10 total visits), whereas about one-third of the sample was recommended for weekly home visiting (16–20 total visits), and the rest were recommended for monthly visits (4–6 total visits). On average, families were receptive to these levels of home visiting, participating in a majority of the recommended levels. Specific rates of recommendation and participation for grades 2–5 are shown in Table 4.4.

## Profiles of Participation

In an attempt to better understand patterns of participation across the different components of the Fast Track intervention (school-based services, extracurricular groups, home visits), Nix, Pinderhughes, Bierman, Maples, and CPPRG (2005) conducted a latent profile analysis to identify different profiles of family participation in school-based services, extracurricular groups (Parent Groups and Friendship Groups), and home visits. Four profiles of participation emerged. Forty-nine percent of the sample fell into a profile class that was characterized by a high level of participation in all intervention services, receiving an average of 92%, 88%, and 92% of school-based services, extracurricular

**TABLE 4.4. Participation in Home Visiting in Grades 2–5**

| | Weekly | | Biweekly | | Monthly | |
|---|---|---|---|---|---|---|
| Grade level | % recommended | % attended | % recommended | % attended | % recommended | % attended |
| Grade 2 | 34 | 82 | 50 | 71 | 15 | 62 |
| Grade 3 | 31 | 89 | 51 | 71 | 18 | 61 |
| Grade 4 | 25 | 85 | 48 | 78 | 27 | 64 |
| Grade 5 | 25 | 80 | 48 | 75 | 27 | 60 |

*Note.* In grades 2–5, families were recommended for varying levels of home visiting during the school year, depending upon family functioning and need for intervention. Recommended levels were weekly (16–20), biweekly (8–10), and monthly (4–6).

groups, and home visits, respectively. A smaller, but notable proportion of the sample (35%) showed a profile characterized by participation in fewer school-based services and extracurricular groups (78% and 60%, respectively) but higher levels of home visits (averaging 134% of the recommended levels). A small number of children and families (10% of the sample) participated in low levels of each component of Fast Track, and an even smaller group (6% of the sample) participated in more than the recommended levels of intervention (96% of school-based services, 97% of therapeutic groups, and 266% of recommended home visits).

## CASE STUDIES

The two case studies provide an example of how individual families navigated the intervention services provided by Fast Track during the elementary school years.

### *Jeremiah and Grace Locke*

Throughout the elementary school phase of Fast Track, Jeremiah and his mother Grace were very engaged. In first and second grade, Jeremiah participated in over 75% of planned services, which included a Friendship Group, peer pairing, and academic tutoring. Similarly, Grace attended most (60%) of the Parent Group sessions. By third grade, things were going better for Jeremiah in school and he no longer needed tutoring or peer pairing. Although he and his mother attended only a few group sessions in third grade, they both attended a majority of the group sessions in fourth and fifth grades. In addition to Parent Group, Grace was extremely engaged in home visiting during the elementary school years. Although she qualified

for biweekly home visits based on the FC's ratings of family functioning, she received extra support, with visits occurring weekly
on average. Grace was interested in additional home visits because
she continued to argue frequently with Jeremiah. She had trouble
getting Jeremiah to do what she asked and found this frustrating.
Grace would shout at and threaten Jeremiah, who would yell and
hit. During home visits, the FC worked with Grace to help her find
alternative ways to deal with Jeremiah's defiance and to continue to
talk with him. As Jeremiah got older, he and Grace participated in
the middle school transition program components. Overall, despite
her continuing parenting challenges, Grace felt that the school components of Fast Track were very helpful to Jeremiah, and greatly
appreciated the parenting support she received.

### Cindy and Susan Steele

During the elementary phase of Fast Track, Cindy participated fully.
She frequently attended Friendship Group and peer-pairing sessions
throughout the elementary school years and received almost all of
the planned tutoring sessions each year, as well. Susan attended a
majority of the Parent Group sessions during the elementary years,
participating in an average of 70% of the sessions each year. However, Susan was less interested in home visits, completing fewer than
half of the biweekly home visits recommended for her throughout
the elementary school years. Her FC observed that Susan was reluctant to utilize the positive parenting strategies she learned in Parent
Group, and Susan expressed concerns that the strategies were not
very helpful in managing Cindy's defiant behavior at home. Overall,
Susan continued to be overwhelmed by high levels of stress in her
life. Along with the challenges of raising her four children, Susan
was coping with financial and legal problems, stressed by the high
level of drug-related crimes in her neighborhood, and troubled by
medical problems. Susan felt mixed about the impact of Fast Track.
On the one hand, she was satisfied with the benefits of the Fast
Track services that Cindy received, but on the other she still found
it challenging to manage Cindy's behavior at home.

## STUDIES OF FAST TRACK IMPLEMENTATION

Three kinds of studies were undertaken to better understand Fast Track
intervention participation in the elementary years. These studies focused
on (1) child, family, and contextual factors that predicted the amount
and quality of intervention participation; (2) the degree to which different dimensions of intervention participation predicted child and parent

outcomes; and (3) evaluation of the utility of the strategies used to tailor participation levels in the home-visiting and peer-pairing components of the intervention.

## Predicting Intervention Participation

In an initial study, we examined the degree to which site, child characteristics, and family characteristics predicted participation in the school-based intervention components, the extracurricular groups, and the home-visiting component of Fast Track (Nix et al., 2005). For the school-based intervention components, the only significant predictor was site. Child participation in the school-based intervention components was highest in the small, stable school districts of rural Pennsylvania, and lowest in the large, highly mobile school districts at the Seattle site (with Nashville and Durham participation rates intermediate in level). Participation in the extracurricular groups (Parent Groups and Friendship Groups) was also highest at the Pennsylvania site and also predicted by parent age, exposure to higher levels of stressful life events, and being white (rather than black). Most likely, these site effects reflect differences in the mobility of the families served and the nature and dynamics at schools that impeded or facilitated service delivery by Fast Track ECs. In contrast, participation in home visits did not differ across sites, but varied as a function of family characteristics. Lower family SES, being black (rather than white), being a single parent, having higher levels of depressive symptoms, living in an especially poor neighborhood, and having a child with lower IQ all predicted higher levels of home visit participation. In general, the amount of variance accounted for by these predictors was quite small: 12% for the school-based components, 13% for the extracurricular groups, and 16% for home visits. The fact that intervention participation was generally high and was not highly affected by child, family, or contextual factors likely reflects the success of efforts made by Fast Track staff to remove barriers to participation and to deliver services to all families.

A second study examined a somewhat different question by focusing on the degree to which child, family, or contextual factors affected the quality of (rather than attendance at) Parent Group sessions during the first-grade year (Nix et al., 2009.) Prior research suggested that family risk factors often undermine the quality of parental participation in intervention (Baydar, Reid, & Webster-Stratton, 2003; Dumas et al., 2007). Using hierarchical linear models in which families were nested in Parent Groups, we showed similar effects in Fast Track. Higher FC ratings of the quality of parent participation were predicted by having a spouse or long-term partner (vs. being a single parent), being older, having more education, having a more prestigious job, being less depressed, having a better home environment, living in a better neighborhood, being white (vs. black), and having a child with less severe behavior problems at school. Interestingly, intraclass correlation coefficients also revealed that the specific groups parents were part of significantly affected the quality of their participation, accounting for 22% of the variance after all other factors were considered. This finding is consistent with another Fast Track study that suggested that some FCs (and some Parent Groups) were more effective than others (Orrell-Valente et al., 1999). In the Orrell-Valente and colleagues study, we found that the degree of trust and positive working alliance that FCs built with each family predicted the quality of parent engagement and participation in intervention services. In addition, we found that the greater the similarity between parent and FC background characteristics and experiences (such as ethnic match), the more likely they would have a more positive therapeutic working alliance.

We also explored the predictors of the quality of child participation in first-grade Friendship Groups (Lavallee, Bierman, Nix, & CPPRG, 2005). Again, using hierarchical linear models that accounted for the nesting of children within Friendship Groups, we found that children's baseline (preintervention) behavior was an important predictor of their behavior during Friendship Group sessions. Not surprisingly, children who were the hardest to manage in the classroom were most likely to show the lowest levels of positive participation and elevated levels of negative behavior during Friendship Group sessions. In general, once the influence of the child's baseline behavior on their in-session behavior was accounted for, the behavioral characteristics of their peer partners did not add explanatory value to their level of positive participation and level of negative behavior. The one exception was a group effect in which the average peer-partner baseline aggression levels predicted lower levels of child in-session positive engagement. This finding suggests that placing highly aggressive children together in a group can reduce the quality of child participation.

## Associations between Intervention Participation and Outcomes

We also examined the relationship between intervention participation and outcomes, for both parents and children. Focusing on parents, we found that how often parents attended Parent Group during first grade was unrelated to intervention outcomes (Nix et al., 2009). However, the *quality* of parent participation did predict positive changes in parental perceptions of their children, parental warmth, reduced use of physical punishment, and higher levels of involvement with the child's school by the end of the first-grade year. The particular FC and group that a parent was assigned to also made a difference, predicting 14% of the variance in parental warmth and 16% of the variance in school involvement. As noted above, by employing extensive supports (transportation, snacks, payment to parents), Fast Track was able to encourage high levels of attendance at Parent Groups, even when family risks may otherwise have kept families away. However, attendance alone was not enough to optimize positive intervention outcomes. Better outcomes emerged when parents participated actively in the intervention sessions. To some degree, the amount of change was a function of the quality of the specific groups (or FCs) parents were assigned to, but higher levels of family risk factors also decreased high-quality participation. Mediation analyses suggested that lower SES (i.e., parent education and parent occupation) was associated with reduced intervention effects on parenting at the end of first grade primarily because it was associated with lower-quality participation in the Parent Groups.

These findings have several implications for the design of parenting interventions, particularly when these programs are designed to serve parents with multiple risk factors, as in the case of Fast Track. First, improving the quality of parent participation in Parent Group sessions appears critical to optimizing benefits for parents. This may require modifications to the educational format used in Fast Track and most other parent management training programs in order to more effectively engage parents with less education and who are living under conditions of considerable hardship. Careful attention to the characteristics of the group leader and group composition may also be needed to increase high-quality parent participation (see also Robbins, Turner, Alexander, & Perez, 2003). Certainly, a better understanding of the factors associated with producing strong working alliances and positive Parent Group participation levels might inform intervention design and help improve the selection and training of effective FCs. In addition, the Fast Track findings suggest that a subset of families (i.e., single parents, low SES, black) tended to prefer individualized home visits rather than Parent Group sessions. By supplementing the therapeutic groups with individualized home visits, Fast Track was able to reach these children and parents who might not have received services otherwise. Hence, providing the option of Parent Group versus individual (home visit) sessions may be another strategy that can increase the active engagement of multirisk parents in preventive interventions. Interestingly, a meta-analysis of parent management training effects suggests that socially and economically disadvantaged parents may do better with individually focused parent management training than with group-based approaches (Lundahl, Risser, & Lovejoy, 2006).

We also explored links between the quality of Friendship Group participation and child outcomes (Lavallee et al., 2005). Several researchers have raised concerns about grouping aggressive children together due to the possibility that negative peer influences during intervention sessions may have iatrogenic effects because they model aggressive behavior or positively reinforce it with laughter or imitation (Dishion & Tipsord, 2011). In addition, aggressive children are particularly likely to react negatively to conflict during cooperative peer activities and escalate conflicts, as they attempt to dominate rather than resolve disagreements (Asarnow, 1983). Additional research has suggested that aggressive behavior becomes more acceptable to children when it is displayed by a majority of group members (Boivin, Dodge, & Coie, 1995; Wright et al., 1986). Our analyses of Fast Track Friendship Groups in the early elementary grades showed that child behavior in group sessions (high rates of positive in-session behavior and low rates of negative in-session behavior) predicted improvements in teacher-rated and observed prosocial behavior and aggression (Lavallee et al., 2005). When peer partners provided attention and reinforcement for a child's disruptive activities during Friendship Group sessions, less improvement was evident in postintervention levels of peer-nominated and teacher-rated aggression. Interestingly, a higher proportion of girls in a particular Friendship Group emerged as an important group characteristic, significantly predicting greater gains in teacher and peer-nominated prosocial behavior, as well as greater reductions in aggression for both boys and girls.

In general, our findings suggest that groups of aggressive children can often be managed effectively and provide an effective context for social skill training. In most of the Fast Track groups, children participated with positive behaviors and exhibited minimal conflict, and these in-session behaviors predicted positive behavioral outcomes. However, about 20% of the time, groups were challenging to manage, and 5% of the time child behavior was significantly problematic in the Friendship Group context and peer deviancy training was evident. In these cases, poor-quality child participation and negative peer escalation undermined intervention benefits. It appears, however, that such unintended consequences can be minimized by avoiding groups in which the most aggressive children are placed together, integrating girls with boys, including nonaggressive children in the groups, and carefully monitoring group processes during the course of intervention. It also may be worthwhile to consider alternative effective strategies—such as creating smaller groups, conducting shorter intervention sessions, and providing individual coaching—to improve the behavioral adjustment of the very aggressive children in social skill training programs (Bierman, 2004).

## Utility of the Adaptive Intervention Components in the Elementary Years

With the advent of tailored, "personalized" approaches to preventive intervention design, there is great interest in, but relatively little research on, how best to implement tailoring strategies (Collins, Murphy, & Bierman, 2004). After first grade, Fast Track began to tailor some of the components as needed for families (frequency of home visits) and thus could begin to investigate this issue. In one study, we examined the utility of the adaptive intervention components, focusing on the validity of the assessments used to tailor levels of home visits.

Fast Track tailored levels of home visits in grades 2–5 in order to provide a dose that we hypothesized would most effectively and efficiently meet the needs of different families. To do so, Fast Track had FCs complete a brief rating scale designed to assess the variations in parental functioning and family stressors (parenting skills, parental well-being, and parent–school involvement) that indicated differential need for home visits. In addition, FCs and their supervisors were allowed to use their clinical judgment to take into consideration extenuating circumstances that might increase or decrease the level of home visiting needed by a particular family indicated by the rating scale. Analyses of these measures indicated that the FC ratings of family functioning were reasonably reliable and provided incremental validity in predicting children's school behavioral outcomes beyond baseline, research-based measures of family functioning (Bierman, Nix, Maples, Murphy, & CPPRG, 2006). In contrast, global judgments made by FCs about family need were vulnerable to biases associated with site, child sex, and race. These findings are consistent with other research suggesting that therapists are relatively good at providing sensitive descriptions of client functioning using standardized rating scales, but less good at synthesizing multiple pieces of information to form one global, categorical assessment of treatment need (Westen & Weinberger, 2004).

To assess the impact of the Fast Track tailoring of home visits on intervention impact, a set of weighted regression analyses was used to simulate and compare parent and child outcomes under three hypothetical implementation conditions: (1) using research-based measures alone to tailor levels of home visiting, (2) using FCs' ratings of parental functioning to set dose recommendations, and (3) examining the impact of the intervention as conducted (e.g., setting the dose of home visits based on clinical ratings of parental functioning but allowing deviations based on global assessments of family need) (Bierman et al., 2006). Our findings suggested that the strongest impact on child third-grade school behavior problems occurred in the second condition, when FC ratings of family functioning (alone) were used to tailor levels of home visiting. These analyses suggest that tailoring home visits was useful in Fast Track and could have been optimized by using FC ratings of family functioning to recommend levels of home visits, without allowing FCs and supervisors to make changes to recommended levels. Future research focused on the development of reliable and valid rating scales that could be used to tailor dose recommendations in preventive interventions like Fast Track would be very useful.

## SUMMARY

Fast Track represents one of the first attempts to take a prevention science approach to the next level, by creating a science-based intervention with multiple levels (universal and indicated prevention components), and multiple stakeholders within a community (interfacing with schools, families, and community service and youth agencies.) Based on a developmental model of early-starting CD, Fast Track started early and addressed multiple skill domains of the child, and sought to support positive development across multiple years and key developmental transitions. The intervention targeted skills in several domains (social, emotional, behavioral, academic) and incorporated multiple support systems, with prevention activities targeting positive behavioral support at school and at home and fostering productive home–school relationships. Overall, Fast Track was implemented as planned, with the exception of the volunteer mentoring program, where it was difficult to recruit the desired number of volunteers.

Several key lessons were learned in the context of the elementary school program delivery. First, high-quality implementation was strongest during the first two elementary years (grades 1–2), when most families remained in core schools and service areas, and when each of the components was delivered with intensity following manualized, evidence-based programs. Over time, several factors led to some fragmentation in the implementation quality of Fast Track. Due primarily to family mobility, participation gradually decreased somewhat across the elementary years. Although Fast Track sought to deliver services within a wide geographical area, modifications in program implementation were necessary when families moved long distances and matriculated at new school districts that were not Fast Track partners. Second, during the less intensive "maintenance" phase (grades 3–5), the monthly group schedule reduced opportunities for focused efforts at supporting parent and child skill acquisition. The value of these boosters remains unclear. Increasingly, the Fast Track intervention became more individualized over time, and several elements (academic tutoring, homework club, social club, home visiting) were delivered following general guidelines rather than standardized manuals. We could track rates of participation in those program components, but the quality was harder to discern because the program was delivered in more flexible ways across sites and staff. This may have reduced impact. The mobility of the Fast Track sample and the increasing levels of individualization and flexibility in several intervention components led to reduced levels of participation over time and likely also to reduced (or more variable) implementation quality.

Second, our analyses revealed the substantial impact of both parent and child intervention participation quality on later outcomes. Fast Track devoted considerable resources to, and was quite successful in attaining, good intervention participation rates. However, quality of participation still varied considerably across individual parents and children, which proved to be a key predictor of intervention benefit. Hence, additional attention to promoting high-quality participation in intervention might strengthen program impact.

Finally, important lessons were learned regarding the tailored, adaptive elements of the program. Our analyses suggested that using clinical judgment to make decisions regarding levels and types of additional services needed by individual families and children could be effective—when intervention staff were asked to complete standard ratings regarding participant functioning that were linked with levels of recommended service. At the same time, later analyses suggested that, when intervention staff were allowed to make more global judgments about child or family need for services, these judgments were quite vulnerable to the effects of site and intervention staff biases that reduced their reliability and validity. Hence, Fast Track would have been better off to use just the standardized staff ratings and cutoffs to determine levels of individualized services, rather than also allowing intervention staff and supervisors to make changes to these service recommendations.

# Chapter 5

# Impact of the Fast Track Intervention during the Elementary School Years

This chapter describes the initial impact of the Fast Track intervention on children during elementary school (i.e., grades 1–5). We describe the impact on the children and parents receiving Fast Track services first, followed by the impact of the universal Fast Track intervention services on classmates who did not receive additional services. The results we present represent "intent-to-treat" findings (Brown, 1993), which compare the outcomes of all families who were randomly assigned to the intervention and comparison groups. These findings are likely to be conservative estimates of the impact of the intervention because they incorporate the fact that not all families participated fully in the intervention. As noted in Chapter 3, none of the parents and children entered the study seeking intervention; they volunteered simply to take part in a developmental study and were not offered intervention until later, depending upon the child's first-grade school assignment. However, by including all families assigned to the intervention group in these analyses, the intent-to-treat approach used here protects the randomized design from any selection biases that might occur if we included only those families who were highly motivated and able to participate fully in the intervention.

Although we report intervention effects as if they could be attributed to a particular component (e.g., reading outcomes are attributed to tutoring), because the intervention combined multiple components, we acknowledge that it is not possible to isolate the causal impact of one component versus another on outcomes.

## INITIAL INTERVENTION IMPACT ON CHILDREN AND PARENTS DURING ELEMENTARY SCHOOL

Following from the developmental model presented in Chapter 2, the first 2 years of Fast Track provided intensive intervention support focused on building child social-emotional competencies and positive peer relationships, fostering early academic skills, and promoting positive parenting skills. We anticipated that intensive intervention targeting these early protective factors would boost child functioning by grade 3 and reduce levels of conduct problems and corresponding risk for future antisocial behavior. In grades 3–5, the Fast Track protocol reduced the intensity of group interventions to monthly sessions, and provided individually tailored levels of other intervention components (home visiting, academic tutoring). We provide a summary of child and family outcomes during these elementary years below; a complete report of Fast Track findings is available in papers describing outcomes in first (CPPRG, 1999a), third (CPPRG, 2002a, 2002b), and fourth and fifth (CPPRG, 2002b, 2004a) grades.

### Social-Emotional Competencies

At the end of first grade, after 1 year of intensive programming, children in the Fast Track intervention group showed significant improvement in the social-emotional skills targeted in PATHS and Friendship Groups, with effect sizes ranging from 0.23 to 0.54. Relative to children in the control group, they could more accurately identify emotions and generate appropriate responses for managing strong feelings. The intervention improved their capacity to cope effectively with social difficulties, and children offered more adaptive solutions to problems involving social entry and conflict resolution and generated fewer aggressive responses. Improved social problem-solving skills were still evident at the end of grade 3, and in addition, by the end of grade 3 children in the intervention group reported fewer hostile attributions.

Analyses in grades 4 and 5 documented sustained intervention benefits in the areas of social cognition and social competence, with an effect size of 0.18 (CPPRG, 2004a). Some effects reemerged at grade 4, including a significant intervention impact on peer social preference on the sociometric surveys (CPPRG, 2002b). To understand the potential clinical value of these improvements, we used a "caseness" approach (i.e., a cutoff was set at one $SD$ above the mean of the normative sample for each domain of interest) to assess child social-emotional functioning in grades 4 and 5 (CPPRG, 2004a). By the end of elementary school, Fast Track produced an absolute 7% reduction in the likelihood that high-risk children would emerge as cases with problems in the domain of social functioning (i.e., 23% of control cases vs. 16% of intervention cases). Thus, Fast Track produced a 30% relative reduction in child risk for problematic outcomes in social functioning.

Improved peer relations were also evident by the end of grade 1 (CPPRG, 1999a). Unbiased observers documented higher rates of pro-social peer interaction in the school context for children in the intervention group, and they showed greater gains in peer acceptance reflected in classroom sociometric surveys (effect sizes = 0.27 and 0.28, respectively). These sociometric improvements were not still evident at grade 3 (CPPRG, 2002a). It is possible the sociometric effects faded when peer pairing was discontinued after grade 2; peer pairing provided regular opportunities for positive interactions with normative classmates and may have boosted program impact on the peer perceptions and peer reputations of target children (Bierman, 1986). In addition, between grades 1 and 3, a substantial number of high-risk children moved to different schools and had to adapt to new peer groups. It might be the case that new classmates needed the opportunity to interact positively with these high-risk children in order not to be turned off by what still remained of their aggressive and disruptive behavior. It is also the case that the dispersion of high-risk participants to new schools by grade 3 led to much more missing data on the sociometric measures than on other measures (as we did not have permission to conduct sociometric interviews with each child in the new schools that Fast Track children moved to), and this dispersion may have reduced their utility for assessing intervention impact.

Grade 4 marked the first time at which deviant peer involvement was measured, assessing the degree to which target children were friends with youth who engaged in antisocial activities. By the end of grade 4, children in the intervention group reported less deviant behavior by friends than children in the control group, including lower rates of friends carrying weapons, stealing, using marijuana, and police involvement (CPPRG, 2002b). The caseness analysis conducted at the end of elementary school (grades 4 and 5) revealed a significant absolute reduction of 6% in the likelihood that high-risk children would emerge as cases with problems in the domain of deviant peer involvement (i.e., 18% of control cases vs. 12% of intervention cases) (CPPRG, 2004a). Thus, Fast Track produced a 33% relative reduction in child risk for problematic outcomes in terms of deviant peer involvement (Figure 5.1).

According to the developmental model underlying the Fast Track intervention, one consequence of children's rejection by their peer group in elementary school is an increased likelihood of becoming involved in deviant peer groups as they approach adolescence. Perhaps because of

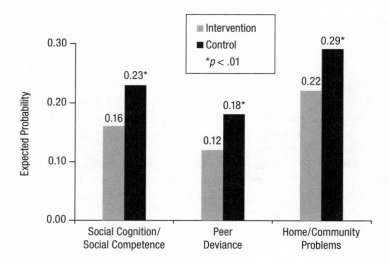

**FIGURE 5.1.** Expected probability of intervention and control children classified as "cases" across domains in grades 4 and 5. Data from CPPRG (2004).

their greater acceptance by their peers in earlier years (CPPRG, 1999a), and because of the intervention's ongoing focus on enhancing children's awareness of the consequences for their actions and on decision-making skills, children receiving the Fast Track intervention may have been better able to avoid involvement with deviant peers during the fourth and fifth grade.

## Academic Skills and School Adjustment

In the academic domain, the first year of intensive academic tutoring promoted positive intervention effects on emergent literacy skills, including the ability to sound out initial and ending sounds, and early word decoding (effect size = 0.56) (CPPRG, 1999a). Reflecting reading skill acquisition, first-grade language arts grades also showed significant benefits for children receiving the Fast Track intervention (effect size = 0.29). Unfortunately, however, these positive effects on academic functioning were no longer evident at the end of grade 3 (CPPRG, 2002a). After first grade, tutoring was provided only to children who fell in the bottom third of the distribution in their reading ability relative to classmates. Most children graduated out of the Wallach and Wallach (1976) phonics-based evidence-based reading program by the end of first grade, and for those who received tutoring in later years, sessions focused on homework completion and test preparation. It is possible that the academic tutoring conducted in later years was not as effective as the manualized program used in first grade. Alternatively (or in addition), it may have been the case that the criteria used to identify children as being "in need" of academic tutoring were faulty. Given the Fast Track design, it is not possible to determine exactly why academic benefits diminished to nonsignificance by grade 3.

However, by the end of grade 3, intervention-group children showed lower levels of teacher-rated conduct problems than control-group children, suggesting a positive impact of Fast Track on child school adjustment. At the end of grade 4, teachers rated intervention children as more improved over the course of the year in academic competence (CPPRG, 2002b). However, the analyses undertaken at the end of elementary school (grades 4 and 5) revealed no significant intervention effects in either the caseness or continuous variables analyses assessing academic and behavioral outcomes in the school setting (CPPRG, 2004a). The failure of Fast Track to produce an effect on school outcomes in the latter years of elementary school was unexpected. The results raise the concern that, even with a very comprehensive, multicomponent, multiyear program, short-term gains in academic performance and school behavioral adjustment of very high-risk children produced by very intensive intervention at school entry may fade as intervention supports are reduced.

## Positive Parenting Practices

By the end of the first year of intervention, intervention-group parents were demonstrating higher levels of warm and positive parenting behaviors and using more appropriate and consistent discipline strategies than were control-group parents, as assessed during semi-structured home observations (CPPRG, 1999a). Relative to the control-group families, they also reported less use of physical punishment in response to hypothetical child misbehavior vignettes and described significant improvements in their capacity to use positive discipline strategies (e.g., state clear expectations, follow through with consequences). Along with these improvements in parenting behaviors, intervention-group parents also reported greater parenting satisfaction and ease of parenting over the course of the year. In addition, teachers reported that intervention parents had greater parental involvement in school. These changes are consistent with the focus of the Fast Track Parent Group sessions and home visits. Effect sizes ranged from 0.23 to 0.70.

Most of these positive intervention effects on parenting practices were sustained through third grade (CPPRG, 2002a). At the end of third grade, intervention-group parents reported more positive changes in their parenting than did control-group parents (effect size = 0.20), and were less likely to use harsh physical punishment in response to hypothetical child misbehavior vignettes (effect size = 0.19). However, effects on teacher reports of parent involvement at school had faded to nonsignificance. It is possible that effects on school involvement were stronger in first grade because school support was a prominent feature of the first-grade Parent Group curriculum, and teachers visited first-grade Parent Groups. Parents also may have been more responsive to suggestions that they get involved in school when their children were younger and in the process of making the important school transition into first grade.

Overall, parents continued to report high levels of satisfaction with the Fast Track intervention at the end of third grade. They appreciated the help provided to them and their children through the various intervention components, and also reported that Fast Track was helpful to other children in the family. Although Fast Track included no independent assessments of the functioning of nontarget siblings in third grade, these parent-report data are consistent with findings reported by others who have used family-based interventions (e.g., Humphreys, Forehand, McMahon, & Roberts, 1978). It may be that the home-visiting component was especially facilitative of such effects, given that one of its primary goals was to assist parents in generalizing their newly acquired parenting skills from the Parent Group and Parent–Child Sharing time to the home.

## Conduct Problems and Antisocial Behavior

A central aim of Fast Track was to reduce serious conduct problems exhibited in home and school settings, including physical aggression, stealing, substance use, and engaging in arson or property destruction. According to the conceptual model guiding the Fast Track intervention design, gains in the targeted child and parent competencies in the first 2 years should, over time, promote reductions in child conduct problems. One measure suggested some initial intervention effects on child conduct problems at the end of the first year of intervention: Unbiased observers documented significant reductions in disruptive behavior at school (effect size = 0.31) (CPPRG, 1999a). In addition, both parents and teachers rated intervention-group children as showing greater reductions in conduct problems than control-group children compared to their behavior before Fast Track began (effect sizes = 0.50 and 0.53, respectively). However, neither parent nor teacher ratings indicated significant intervention effects on actual rates of conduct problems at the end of grade

1, nor did behavioral observations conducted at home significantly favor the intervention group. One likely explanation for these findings is that the intervention-group children may have made small but significant progress in this area but continued to exhibit sufficiently disruptive behavior that parents and teachers still viewed them as problematic.

However, by the end of third grade, the gap between intervention- and control-group children had widened, and children in the intervention group were significantly less likely to exhibit serious conduct problems (CPPRG, 2002a). Specifically, at the end of grade 3, teachers reported significantly lower rates of child aggressive, disruptive, and disobedient behaviors for the intervention-group children (effect size = 0.19). Parents of intervention-group children also reported significantly fewer problem behaviors on the Parent Daily Report measure (effect size = 0.15), although they did not report fewer conduct problem symptoms in diagnostic interviews. In addition, both parents and teachers rated intervention-group children as showing greater reductions in conduct problems than control-group children (effect sizes = 0.20 and 0.27, respectively).

Because the goal of this prevention trial was to lower the incidence rates of serious conduct problems, the true test of prevention effectiveness is not just to document mean changes in the overall level of problem behavior in the intervention sample, but also to lower the incidence rate of cases of CD in that sample. To test whether Fast Track was reducing cases of CD, we devised a multisource index of serious conduct problems (i.e., clinical caseness) (CPPRG, 2002a). Clinical caseness was based on the presence of an elevated score on at least one of the following measures: (1) a Diagnostic Interview Schedule for Children (DISC) diagnosis of ODD or CD, (2) existence of an individualized education plan (IEP), and (3) teacher or parent reports of conduct problems in the top 15% of the distribution. Note that given the methods for identifying the high-risk sample in kindergarten described earlier (i.e., very high elevations on parent and/or teacher reports of conduct problems), none of the high-risk sample were "case-free" prior to the start of the intervention. Using this person-oriented approach to data analysis revealed that 37% of the intervention sample was "case free" at the end of grade 3, in contrast to only 27% of the control sample. This difference represents a clinically significant 37% increase in "case-free" status associated with the Fast Track intervention (Figure 5.2).

Reductions in parent-reported and child-reported behavior problems (in this case, as a combined measure) for Fast Track intervention-group children, relative to control-group children, continued to be maintained through grades 4 and 5, with an effect size of 0.15 (CPPRG, 2004a). The caseness analysis conducted at the end of elementary school (grades 4 and 5) showed a significant absolute reduction of 7% in the

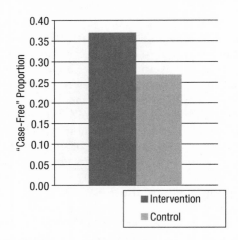

**FIGURE 5.2.** Proportion of intervention and control children classified as "case-free" in grade 3. From CPPRG (2002a, p. 30). Copyright © 2002 Plenum Publishing Corporation. Reprinted with permission from Springer.

likelihood that high-risk children would emerge as cases with problems in the domain of conduct problems in home and community settings (i.e., 29% of control cases vs. 22% of intervention cases) (CPPRG, 2004a). Thus, Fast Track produced a 32% relative reduction in child risk for problematic outcomes in terms of conduct problems in home and community settings.

Compared to control-group children, fewer Fast Track children engaged in serious levels of parent-rated aggressive behavior and self-reported delinquent behavior and substance use during the fourth- and fifth-grade years. The lower rate of serious levels of conduct problems in the home and community during the final years of elementary school suggested that the developmental course toward serious antisocial behavior may have been substantially altered, at least for some Fast Track children.

## Summary

Analyses at the end of first grade documented support for the early effectiveness of the Fast Track intervention in promoting children's social-emotional understanding and competencies, positive peer relations, and reading skills, and fostering more warm-responsive parent–child interactions and the use of positive discipline practices. By third grade, reductions in conduct problems were evident in school and home settings (see

CPPRG, 1999a, 2002a, for more details). Effect sizes for program outcomes were modest, but we found meaningful reductions in the number of children exhibiting clinically significant levels of impairment.

In the arenas of social-emotional competence and peer relations, parenting practices, and conduct problems in the home and community, the findings in grades 4 and 5 indicate that the Fast Track program produced modest improvement that was sustained through the end of elementary school, supporting prior indications of the Fast Track program's effectiveness through grade 3. More importantly, these findings demonstrated that Fast Track reduced the risk experienced by children with early-onset conduct problems of becoming involved in serious problems evident at the end of elementary school in grades 4 and 5 (CPPRG, 2004a). Prior preventive intervention projects have demonstrated significant effects on children's conduct problems in early elementary school (e.g., Gross et al., 2003; Walker, Stiller, Severson, Feil, & Golly, 1998), leading to reductions in behavior problems in high-risk children, and these gains have been maintained through follow-up assessments years later. Other preventive interventions delivered at specific points in the elementary school years have also had long-term follow-up effects on children's later serious conduct problems, delinquency, police arrest, and substance use (Eddy, Reid, Stoolmiller, & Fetrow, 2003; Lochman & Wells, 2004; Lochman, Wells, Qu, & Chen, 2013; Tremblay, Pagani-Kurtz, Masse, Vitaro, & Pihl, 1995). However, Fast Track is the first preventive intervention to provide comprehensive intervention components timed throughout the elementary school years with a very high-risk sample, producing changes in at-risk children's social and behavioral functioning throughout that entire period of time. Overall, these elementary school results demonstrate the potential for adapting intervention components originally developed in clinic settings with focused samples and making them suitable for preventive efforts targeting high-risk populations in naturally occurring high-risk communities across a wide cross-section of American contexts.

## TESTS OF INTERVENTION MEDIATION IN THE ELEMENTARY SCHOOL YEARS

We also conducted analyses to test the proposed mechanisms of action underlying the Fast Track intervention and to provide insight regarding the ways in which the Fast Track intervention achieved its outcomes during elementary school. These analyses examined intervention effects on child and parent competencies at the end of grade 3 as mediators of child outcomes at the end of grade 4 (CPPRG, 2002b). We tested three mediators, including improvements during grades 1–3 in child social cognitions and child social competence at school and reductions in parents' harsh physical discipline practices at home. Four key outcomes were examined in grade 4: peer social preference (assessed with peer sociometrics); association with deviant peers (assessed by child self-report); social and academic competence at school (assessed by teacher ratings); and child conduct problems at home (assessed by parent report). The mediation analyses served as a sort of "manipulation check," to test the hypothesis that the Fast Track intervention (i.e., the experimental manipulation) achieved its goals of improving child functioning at grade 4 by increasing competencies targeted at grades 1–3 that are thought to play a causal role in antisocial development (Maggs & Schulenberg, 2001). An array of developmental studies document correlational links between the mediators selected here (e.g., social cognition, social competence, harsh discipline) and child antisocial outcomes in later years (Coie & Dodge, 1998). However, only mediation analyses within a randomized intervention design can test those same hypotheses in a way that supports interpretations of causality.

The mediation analyses revealed that positive effects of the Fast Track intervention on the four grade 4 child outcomes were statistically accounted for by intervening improvements in the identified proximal targets of intervention assessed at grade 3. The pattern of significant partial mediation that emerged reflected within-domain (rather than cross-domain) associations. For example, improved parenting behavior mediated the intervention effect on the child's aggressive behavior at home but not at school. Improvements in the child's social cognitions about peers mediated the intervention on deviant peer associations. Improvements in prosocial behavior in the school setting mediated intervention effects on classroom peer social preference.

The lack of mediation of the teacher-reported improvement in fourth-grade social competence is just as important as the findings already noted. This variable assessed the teacher's judgment of how much improvement the child made in socially competent behavior between the beginning and end of the fourth-grade school year. The lack of mediation suggests that the effect of intervention on fourth-grade teacher ratings can be attributed to the ongoing intervention in fourth grade rather than any delayed effect of previous intervention. Thus, continued intervention seemed to exert new effects on child outcomes.

These findings directly support the developmental theory that guided the creation of the Fast Track intervention (CPPRG, 1992). They also suggest that in order to achieve positive outcomes, a program ought to have an impact on the targeted domains. The findings have substantial external validity because of the diverse sample in which they were tested (i.e., a racially and ethnically diverse sample of boys and girls from four highly varied geographic sites).

The findings have implications for the design of preventive interventions, following in the traditions of prevention science (e.g., Cicchetti & Toth, 1998), but they also refine developmental theory. Thus, developmental science and prevention science inform each other (Cichetti & Toth, 1998; Maggs & Schulenberg, 2001). The specific pattern of mediation that was found can be interpreted as support for domain specificity in antisocial development. It was hypothesized that changes in children's social cognitions and/or parenting support in one domain would first have effects on child behavior and adjustment within that domain but would lead to spreading effects in other domains. These findings support the former part of the hypothesis to a greater degree than the latter part. These patterns do suggest that a multifaceted intervention may be necessary in order to broadly improve children's adjustment outcomes in the elementary years.

## TESTS OF INTERVENTION MODERATION
## IN THE ELEMENTARY SCHOOL YEARS

In addition to testing for the main effects of the Fast Track intervention during the elementary school years, we conducted additional analyses to determine whether the intervention was differentially effective for particular subgroups with different preintervention characteristics. We examined moderation by demographic variables (e.g., sex, race, site, cohort), child variables (e.g., IQ), family variables (e.g., marital status, SES, parent mental health or substance abuse status), and neighborhood variables (e.g., poverty, instability, quality). Only a few, scattered moderation effects emerged. For example, at the end of first grade, one interaction effect emerged with child sex, indicating that intervention reduced special education involvement for boys but not for girls. However, sex did not moderate other intervention effects, nor was there any indication that the intervention was differentially effective across race, sites, or cohorts.

The few scattered moderation effects in the elementary school analyses did not form any meaningful pattern, and did not extend beyond chance levels. This failure to find systematic evidence of moderation suggests that the modest intervention effects were generalizable during elementary school, with comparable effects, for example, for boys and girls, for black and white children, and in urban and rural settings.

However, one moderation effect related to the effects of the reading tutoring intervention in grade 1 warrants attention. As noted above, intervention had a main effect on reading achievement scores at the end of grade 1 (CPPRG, 1999a), but there was variation in response. Intervention had substantial benefits for children with early reading difficulties who were not inattentive and modest reading achievement benefits for inattentive children without early reading difficulties; however, it had no impact for children who were both inattentive and poor early readers (Rabiner, Malone, & CPPRG, 2004). Perhaps the intervention was not intensive enough for students with co-occurring reading and attention problems.

## CASE STUDIES

We turn now to how Jeremiah and Grace and Cindy and Susan were doing during the elementary school phase of intervention. As we noted in the previous chapter, each family engaged in its own unique way with the intervention, particularly the Parent Group and home-visiting components.

### Jeremiah and Grace Locke

During the early elementary school years, Grace frequently felt overwhelmed by many challenges, including illness, ongoing financial problems, and the death of a close friend. With little support from others, including her partner, she found herself feeling alone in raising Jeremiah. The effects of Fast Track were not immediately apparent for Grace and Jeremiah's relationship. Although Jeremiah acted out less and Grace was more affectionate with him, she still yelled at him a lot, much more often than other parents in Fast Track. The tutoring and peer-pairing services helped Jeremiah in school, which he attended regularly, earning grades of Bs and Cs. He was not as aggressive with peers in class and on the playground. Just before fourth grade, Grace and Jeremiah moved in with her relatives, and this provided them with more stability and social support. Their relationship improved. Grace felt more competent in her parenting, with less frustration and anxiety. She was warmer in her interactions with Jeremiah and stopped using harsh physical punishment. In turn, Jeremiah acted out less and listened to Grace more often. Jeremiah was now feeling that Grace tried to understand his feelings even when they disagreed. Jeremiah continued to do well in school, both academically and socially. Reflecting on Jeremiah's and Grace's active participation in Fast Track, these services seemed to support their improvement.

*Cindy, Susan, and Janice Steele*

At the start of first grade, ongoing health, legal, and financial problems beleaguered the family. Cindy had significant problems at home and school. At home, she was often physically aggressive toward her mother and refused to cooperate. Susan responded with daily yelling and threats to spank Cindy. At school, her teacher described Cindy as argumentative, defiant, stubborn, and mean, with little remorse for her mistreatment of peers. She monopolized her teacher's attention. Cindy also struggled with attention problems and learning difficulties in reading and math. Cindy participated actively in all school-based Fast Track services. Her social difficulties were considerable, and she qualified for ongoing social support as well as additional Fast Track tutoring through fourth grade. Cindy's social awareness grew over time, and she became more aware of the negative impact her aggression had on her peers. She made efforts to make friends and was able to use Fast Track support to increase her prosocial behavior and problem-solving skills with peers, although she continued to have difficulties in unstructured settings like the playground and lunchroom. Even with Fast Track tutoring, however, Cindy continued to struggle academically, earning grades of Cs and Ds in most subjects. At home, the financial difficulties and dangerous neighborhood stressors continued to undermine family stability and Susan's parenting, and Susan still escalated to physical punishment with Cindy. These problems reached a crisis point during the later elementary phase of Fast Track, and Susan's sister, Janice, offered to become Cindy's guardian to help out. Susan reached out to her FC, who worked with her and her sister to facilitate the transition of guardianship and to support conjoint planning and family problem solving. Cindy visited her mother and siblings weekly, but was happy to be living with her aunt, who was in a safer and more stable living situation than her mother. During the elementary years, Cindy and her family faced multiple, chronic challenges and stressors. Fast Track services helped Cindy grow socially and emotionally, and they helped Susan reach out to her sister and access more support for Cindy's parenting. Even so, Cindy continued to struggle at school in core areas of learning and in unstructured peer contexts.

## ELEMENTARY SCHOOL:
## UNIVERSAL SAMPLE FINDINGS AT THE END OF GRADE 1

The PATHS curriculum was provided to all children in the intervention schools, not just the high-risk children, and classmates were also involved as peer pairs in the intervention schools. We wondered whether these children would also benefit from the intervention. Hence, we examined the universal preventive effects of Fast Track from grade 1 through grade 3 (CPPRG, 1999b, 2010b). The high-risk target children were removed from these analyses, thus permitting an examination of the intervention effects on the remaining classmates and comparing those attending schools assigned to the intervention versus control conditions.

The results of this universal intervention at the end of first grade provide evidence of its effectiveness in the domains of both aggression and peer relations (CPPRG, 1999b). There were significant effects of the intervention from the viewpoints of children, teachers, and observers. Sociometric nominations for aggressive and hyperactive-disruptive behaviors revealed lower levels of problem behaviors perceived by children in intervention versus control schools (effect sizes = 0.22 for each). Aggregated teacher ratings similarly showed classroom-level reductions in disruptive and aggressive behaviors in intervention versus control schools. Finally, observer ratings documented higher levels of rule following, better classroom atmosphere, and more on-task behavior in intervention classrooms. These findings reflect robust effects of the universal-level prevention activities on classroom behavior with reductions in aggression and increases in self-control and on-task behavior at the end of first grade.

In addition, teacher ratings and direct observations revealed significant intervention effects on positive peer relations and positive classroom climate, as students showed more mutual liking and expressed more positive affect and enthusiasm in the classroom. There were no significant site-by-condition interaction effects in these analyses, indicating no robust differences in intervention effects as a function of rural versus urban school location, percentage of children below the poverty level, or racial composition of the classrooms.

Although intervention effects were found across raters, these effects were modest in size. This may in part be due to the fact that within schools all teachers, independent of personal interest or ability, were assessed. Thus, teachers who were relatively ineffective, showed little enthusiasm, or completed only a portion of the PATHS curriculum were assessed as if they had completed the intervention; no intervention teachers were dropped for poor-quality implementation, high resistance, or providing a low dosage. In this sense, this intent-to-treat trial design may provide the highest level of external validity regarding how this universal intervention might affect a typical, entire school community.

The findings on the effects of quality of implementation and dosage of PATHS lend credence to the outcome effects. We found that the intervention staff's ratings of how well teachers understood concepts, generalized skills outside the curriculum time, and managed their class-room predicted levels of classroom aggression (based on teachers' mean ratings) as well as observers' ratings of the classroom atmosphere. Thus, higher implementation quality was related to lower levels of classroom aggression and higher ratings of classroom atmosphere. As there had been few comprehensive studies on social competence promotion that had examined how both dosage and quality of implementation affect outcomes when these findings were published (Battistich, Schaps, Watson, & Solomon, 1996; Pentz et al., 1990), they indicated that both quantitative and qualitative indices of curriculum implementation should be assessed in future projects.

## ELEMENTARY SCHOOL:
## UNIVERSAL SAMPLE FINDINGS AT THE END OF GRADE 3

Our next analyses examined the effects of the PATHS universal intervention on behavior change for students who received 3 years of the intervention (CPPRG, 2010b). The longitudinal analysis involved 2,937 children who remained in the same intervention or control schools for grades 1, 2, and 3.*

Significant main effects of the intervention were found with mild-to-moderate effect sizes, ranging from 0.10 to 0.40 for all three teacher-rated outcomes (authority acceptance, cognitive concentration, and social competence). In addition, we found significant intervention effects for two of the three peer-rated sociometric outcomes for boys (aggressive and hyperactive-disruptive nominations). Hence, evidence for effectiveness emerged from the viewpoints of two independent sources of information: teachers and peers. These findings reflect consistent but modest effects of the universal-level prevention activities on behavior for children who remained in the same school for 3 years of sustained exposure. The findings are in line with expectations that universal intervention will have mild-to-moderate effects across an entire population (Cuijpers, 2003; Greenberg & Abenavoli, 2017; Hahn et al., 2007). These findings demonstrate, along with effects on social behavior, improved classroom behavior and teacher perceptions of more effective academic engagement, including increased self-control and on-task behavior. As such,

---

* As noted in Chapter 4, the school district reorganization at the Durham site after the second year of the trial led to the subsequent implementation of PATHS as an indicated rather than a school-based universal intervention. Therefore, none of the participants at the Durham site were included in these analyses.

these findings are consistent with a meta-analysis showing significant effects of SEL programs on both behavioral and academic outcomes (Durlak, Weissberg, Dymnicki, Taylor, & Schellinger, 2011).

To determine whether the effects of the universal intervention were moderated by child sex or baseline levels of aggression, we conducted additional analyses that revealed significant moderation of intervention by child baseline levels of aggressive behavior problems and child sex. The PATHS curriculum had a larger impact on reducing aggression in third grade for children who exhibited higher levels of baseline aggression in the fall of first grade (by teacher report) than for children who started school with low levels of aggressive behavior problems.

Classroom rates of aggressive-disruptive behavior show normative declines between first and third grade, as children become socialized into the rules of school. Hence, relatively few children show trajectories of increasing aggression during these years, making it most likely that an intervention affects aggression by decreasing it in children with high initial levels. Peer nominations, in contrast, tend to show relatively stable levels across the early school years. Hence, intervention may affect peer nominations either by reducing nominations among initially aggressive classmates or by suppressing the initiation of peer aggression during the early school years. Boys are more likely than girls to exhibit overt aggression in peer contexts across the elementary school years. Thus, the overall benefits of universal SEL programs on aggressive outcomes do not appear to be limited to children who show high initial rates (although they benefit more, according to teacher ratings) but appear also to promote sustained nonaggressive orientations among boys, in particular (according to peer nominations). In general, the lack of significant intervention effects on peer sociometric nominations for aggression or hyperactivity among girls may reflect the very low base rate of such nominations for girls during the early elementary years (Bierman et al., 2004).

We also explored moderation by site and school disadvantage. Significant effects emerged for school disadvantage (school-level rates of student poverty) as intervention effects were larger for teacher ratings of authority acceptance, cognitive concentration, and social competence in schools that had average socioeconomic disadvantage than in schools with very high disadvantage as measured by student free or reduced-price lunch rates. It should be remembered that the mean level of poverty in the high-disadvantaged schools was approximately 80% of children qualifying for free or reduced lunch. In contrast, the other schools in this study averaged approximately 45% free or reduced lunch eligibility. For comparison purposes, at that time, nationwide figures indicated that the percentage of children eligible for free and reduced lunch was

39.6% nationwide and was 47.3% for the 500 largest American school districts (U.S. Department of Education, National Center for Education Statistics, 2001). Thus, the effects of this universal model appear to be robust for most schools but not for those at the extreme levels of student poverty.

In theory, two types of mechanisms may contribute to the greater effectiveness of this universal SEL program in schools that served student populations comprising average rates of socioeconomically disadvantaged children. One is that it may have been much easier for teachers at less disadvantaged schools to implement the intervention with sustained, high fidelity over the 3 years studied. Supplementary analyses indicated, however, that there were not wide differences in implementation quality that resulted from school disadvantage. This uniformly high fidelity may have been due to the ongoing, proactive technical assistance provided to teachers by ECs. However, as noted earlier, a substantial weakness of this study is there were no unbiased ratings of teachers' fidelity in delivering the lessons, and the ECs who rated the overall implementation quality may have been unreliable. Hughes, Cavell, Meehan, Zhang, and Collie (2005) have argued that SEL programs that require organized lesson planning, generalized support in nonclassroom settings, and coordination with parents may overwhelm teachers who are working in highly stressed contexts and responding to daily student crises. Even when teachers support these efforts, the capacity to sustain the programs in a broad, school-based manner, consistently over multiple years, might be jeopardized by high rates of student and teacher turnover, which disrupts continuity in skill acquisition and generalization. In spite of these processes operating in more disadvantaged schools, our findings show that the universal intervention reduced aggression (according to both teachers and peers) in both high- and low-poverty schools, especially for boys.

Due to the design of the study, students who did not remain in their original schools from grades 1–3 were not tracked longitudinally. The substantial rate of child turnover in the high-risk urban schools (69% in Nashville and 58% in Seattle) raises an important policy issue for the implementation of effective prevention programming. Given such high mobility, it is unlikely that prevention programs will have substantial impact unless they are conducted across entire school districts or at least larger subunits of very large urban districts (Greenberg, 2004). Such rates of student and teacher turnover mean that establishing the full impact of prevention programming will require large-scale designs (Kendziora & Osher, 2016).

Given the high rate of attrition in the urban districts, one might question the external validity of the findings. As a result, analyses were also conducted separately for Pennsylvania, in which 75% of the beginning students were assessed across time. Findings indicated stronger effects in this rural sample, with significant main-effect findings for the three teacher ratings and for all three sociometric nominations for boys and for two of the three nominations for girls. Thus, in the more stable and low-risk schools, effects were stronger and more pervasive.

Overall, these findings indicate the effectiveness that a universal intervention implemented with fidelity can have in altering child social competence and problem behaviors during the first 3 years of school. It is the largest study of its kind indicating the efficacy of school-based, universal interventions during the elementary school years both for the promotion of competence (Elias, 1995) and for the prevention of maladjustment (Grossman et al., 1997; O'Donnell, Hawkins, Catalano, Abbott, & Day, 1995). However, because of the nature of the experimental design, the current findings cannot adequately answer two important questions. First, because the number of years of intervention exposure was not systematically varied, longitudinal analyses cannot differentiate the impact of having 1 year versus more than 1 year of intervention. Second, the design permits us to understand the effects for multiple years of intervention only for those children who remained in their schools for all 3 years. In addition, the absence of more refined measurement of school systems-level processes (e.g., teacher and principal attitudes and behaviors) provides no information on the processes by which school disadvantage influences child outcomes. Future studies that examine the number of years of exposure and fully characterize the implementation environment at multiple levels will be necessary to provide further answers to these central questions regarding school-based processes of change in prevention research (Greenberg, Domitrovich, Weissberg, & Durlak, 2017).

It should be recognized that the Fast Track universal intervention included intensive intervention with high-risk children as an integral part of the overall universal intervention. Although analyses at the end of grade 1 with and without these high-risk children showed similar patterns (CPPRG, 1999b), it is quite possible that effects of the intervention on the non-high-risk children depend on a simultaneous intervention with the high-risk children. Project staff's commitment to work with high-risk children may have reduced teacher stress and increased teacher interest in implementing a universal intervention. Likewise, the improvements in high-risk children that were due to the selected intervention may have improved classroom peer relations among other children. The current study was not designed to evaluate the effects of a universal intervention that excludes simultaneous intensive intervention with a selected group of high-risk children; thus, it does not assess the use of the universal intervention alone. Instead, this study clearly supports the hypothesis that an integrated approach that combines universal and selected intervention can have powerful effects at the universal level of analysis.

## SUMMARY

During elementary school, Fast Track had modest, sustained effects on key domains of functioning for children in the intervention condition. Effect sizes were strongest following the initial, intensive prevention efforts. Mediation analyses indicated that the intervention effects were domain specific (e.g., changes in parenting accounting for child behavior change in the home but not school), thereby indicating the importance of a multicomponent intervention such as Fast Track when dealing with very high-risk children and families. Furthermore, the effects were largely generalizable across child sex and race, site, and cohort.

Because the PATHS curriculum was provided to all of the children in the intervention schools, not just the high-risk children, we also examined the extent to which those children benefitted from the intervention. In first grade, we obtained positive intervention effects for aggression and peer relations for classrooms in which the universal intervention was implemented. Furthermore, the quality of the teachers' implementation of the PATHS curriculum in grade 1 was clearly related to positive outcomes. Additional analyses of behavior change for students who received 3 years of the PATHS intervention provided further support of the curriculum's effects on promoting social competence and reducing aggression.

# Chapter 6

# The Fast Track Intervention in Middle and High School

This chapter describes the early adolescent phase of the Fast Track prevention program (grades 6–10) when children were (on average) 12–16 years old. We first describe the basic organization and structure of the intervention and the staffing arrangements. Then we describe each of the intervention components in more detail, including the rationale for the inclusion of each component and the assessment model used to tailor the prevention services. Finally, we provide implementation data, including amount of participation, along with data on the validity of the tailoring assessments.

Across both early elementary and adolescent phases, the Fast Track prevention program emphasized the promotion of child academic and social-emotional competencies, positive parenting, and school adjustment as protective factors to reduce risk for CD (Dodge et al., 1990). However, there were some notable shifts in the particular content and form of service delivery during the later phase, which were undertaken in recognition of the developmental changes that occur in the developmental progression of CD in adolescence (see model in Chapter 2). Normatively, the frequency of conduct problem behaviors rises during early adolescence, peaking at around age 15–16 and then declining thereafter (Blumstein, Cohen, Roth, & Visher, 1986). In the general population, rates of clinically significant conduct problems double as children move from childhood into adolescence (increasing from 2 to 4% for girls, and from 7 to 15% for boys) (Offord, Boyle, & Racine, 1991). The dramatic increase reflects new, age-related influences that escalate rates of problem behaviors for at-risk adolescents (CPPRG, 2004b; Kimonis, Frick, & McMahon, 2014). In addition, adolescence is also a period of increased onset for other major life problems associated with CD, including substance abuse, major affective disorders, and risky sexual activity.

## ORGANIZATION OF THE ADOLESCENT-PHASE INTERVENTION

Accordingly, the Fast Track prevention model underwent changes as children transitioned into early adolescence (grades 6 and 7) and additional modifications as children moved through adolescence (grades 8–10). These shifts in the Fast Track intervention design were informed by research on risk factors associated with the likelihood of increased antisocial activity during adolescence, as well as protective factors associated with decreased antisocial activity. The intervention also recognized the critical role of addressing the common comorbid difficulties associated with and contributing to antisocial development, particularly substance use and risky sexual activity. As described in more detail in this chapter, the adolescent intervention phase focused on four major domains of youth functioning: (1) academic achievement; (2) peer relations; (3) adult involvement, supervision, and monitoring; and (4) attitudes, identity, values, and beliefs. Parallel to the organization of the elementary intervention, these domains were targeted with a combination of standard program components that were offered to all participating families (e.g., youth and Parent Group sessions, middle school transition program), and other components that were delivered adaptively, with the level and type of service tailored for individual youth based on triannual assessments of child and family functioning and needs.

There were four major differences between the early elementary and adolescent intervention structures. First, the universal (school-based) intervention was discontinued after fifth grade when most children moved into middle schools. At that point in time, children from intervention and control schools merged into the same school, making it impossible to deliver a universal intervention that was received only by youth in the intervention group. Second, relative to the early elementary phase, group-based interventions were de-emphasized in adolescence, in order to reduce risks associated with promoting deviant peer associations (Dishion, McCord, & Poulin, 1999). Standard intervention components delivered to all intervention group youth included parent–youth groups focused on communication, sex education, and substance use prevention in grades 6 and 7 and youth groups focused on identity development and vocational exploration. There was also a standard program designed to provide support at the middle school transition.

Third, individualized prevention planning characterized a larger proportion of the intervention components. Three times per year, intervention staff completed brief assessments of youth risk and protective factors to identify areas of prevention need (e.g., academic achievement; peer relations; adult involvement and monitoring; and attitudes, identity, and values). They then selected from a menu of options to design a prevention action plan composed of individually tailored intervention strategies (Table 6.1).

Finally, the staffing model shifted in the adolescent intervention phase. Intervention staff roles were divided during the elementary phase, with ECs working with children and in the school and FCs working with parents and families. In the adolescent phase, these roles were merged, with one Youth Coordinator (YC) assigned to work with each youth, his or her school, and his or her family. This reorganization reflected the de-emphasis on standard youth and family programming during adolescence, and the increasing emphasis on tailoring intervention activities for youth and their families. These changes phased in over the middle

**TABLE 6.1. Numbers of Sessions of Intervention Components Offered during Grades 6–10**

| Components | Adolescent-phase grade levels | | | | |
| --- | --- | --- | --- | --- | --- |
| | 6 | 7 | 8 | 9 | 10 |
| Standard components | | | | | |
| Parent groups | 7 | — | — | — | — |
| Youth groups | 7 | 4 | 4 | — | — |
| Parent/youth group sessions | 2 | 3 | — | — | — |
| Middle school transition sessions | Varied | — | — | — | — |
| Tailored components | | | | | |
| Family/youth supports | 9–36 | 9–72 | 9–72 | 9–72 | 9–72 |
| Academic support | 0–60 | 0–96 | 0–96 | 0–96 | 0–96 |

Note. Starting in seventh grade, recommended levels and types of tailored intervention components were based on triannual assessments and individual action plans. Table entries reflect the number of contacts. Middle school transition program content was delivered at different times depending upon the timing of youth school transitions.

school transition as group sessions diminished, with two staff members continuing through grade 6, and one staff member continuing thereafter.

## STANDARD FAST TRACK PREVENTION COMPONENTS IN THE ADOLESCENT PHASE

### Parent Groups and Youth Forums

In grade 6, parents and youth spent an increasing amount of group time together in sessions (rather than in separate parent and youth groups), discussing school-transition pressures, boy–girl relationships, vocational interests, and drug and alcohol prevention. In grade 7, parents and youth had three group sessions together, two focused on drug and alcohol prevention, and one focused on vocational interests. Parent Groups were discontinued after grade 7. In grades 7 and 8, youth were offered four workshop sessions (called forums) that addressed vocational opportunities, life skills, and summer employment opportunities. These included four sessions focused on Oyserman, Terry, and Bybee's (2002) school-to-jobs intervention aimed at strengthening emerging identity and building a strong sense of future possibilities and goals (personal selves).

### Middle School Transition Program

The adolescent-phase program began in the spring preceding the child's transition to a higher-level school (from elementary to middle school, or from elementary or middle school to junior high school) and continued through the middle of the following school year. Children transitioned from smaller schools with self-contained classrooms (elementary level) to larger schools with fluid class structures (middle or junior high schools) at different grade levels both across and within the different sites. Although the majority of children in the sample transitioned between grades 5 and 6, substantial subgroups transitioned between grades 4 and 5 or between grades 6 and 7. The program included ten sessions for children and eight sessions for parents. Because various school systems sometimes administered programs similar to this one, this program was altered flexibly to eliminate redundancy with school practices.

We designed the middle school transition program to help youth and their parents adjust to the new demands, opportunities, and risks of the middle school context. At the transition from elementary to middle or junior high school, academic demands increase, as do demands for independent and self-regulated behavioral control and study skills. Socially, the peer group becomes large and diverse, presenting children with new challenges in areas of group entry and peer pressure. The transition program was designed to foster youth coping and adaptation at this important developmental juncture.

The transition program included a set of individual or small-group experiences. These experiences included orientation and tours of the middle school and discussion activities designed to provide support for parents and youth in the weeks immediately preceding and following the transition. In addition, visits from school counselors, experienced parents, and older peers were scheduled during these sessions to provide children and parents with information about what the middle or junior high school would be like. Visits to the middle or junior high school were also scheduled for parents and youth, to provide them with an orientation to the new building and (for youth) with an *in vivo* experience of a typical day at the middle or junior high school building. Older students served as "buddies" for younger students during these visits, providing support and giving information and advice.

In general, the number of group sessions for parents and youth decreased during the early adolescent phase, and were phased out completely after seventh grade (for parents) and after eighth grade (for youth). Prevention services became more individualized during the adolescent phase, following our goal of tailoring the intensity and focus of prevention services to optimally meet individual youth and family needs.

## INDIVIDUALIZED ASSESSMENTS AND INTERVENTION COMPONENTS IN THE ADOLESCENT PHASE

In grades 7–10, YCs completed a triannual assessment three times per year (September, January, May). Based on information gathered from parents, youth, school personnel, staff observations, and any additional input provided by community agencies serving the target youth, YCs rated each youth's risk and protective factors in each of four targeted domains. These ratings were used to determine a risk score in each domain (described in more detail below) that indicated a need for services. YCs then selected services to address those needs from a Fast Track menu and created an individual action plan that was reviewed and updated triennially. The Fast Track menu of possible intervention strategies included seven kinds of prevention activities: family meetings, parent meetings, youth meetings, mentoring sessions, group meetings, academic support, and school/agency consultation. The following sections describe the assessment and intervention focus that characterized each of the four domains of youth functioning in more detail.

## Academic Achievement and Orientation

The secondary schools that Fast Track participants transitioned into during early adolescence were often quite large and required youth to interact with multiple teachers and respond to heightened expectations for independent study and academic attainment. Based on prior research, we anticipated that this transition would contribute to decreased academic self-efficacy and motivation, lower grades, and reduced school engagement for many youth (Brown & Klute, 2003). A key goal of Fast Track was to reduce risks associated with declining academic engagement by helping youth focus on future occupational and employment goals and by addressing school stressors.

The level of youth functioning and degree of risk were assessed on the basis of school grades and academic motivation, as reported by teachers/counselors and reflected in student grades. Failing grades (e.g., Ds and Fs) or recent deterioration in grades, negative attitudes toward school and educational attainment, poor attendance and truancy, and school disciplinary actions were all risk factors; passing grades (Cs and above), a positive commitment toward education and high school completion, and long-term vocational goals were protective factors.

In attempting to improve youths' academic achievement, intervention most often included direct tutoring to remediate skill deficits and to avoid school failure. It also included other strategies designed to foster homework completion, and to promote a positive motivation toward the development of goals and skills for future academic and vocational attainments. Specific prevention strategies on the Fast Track menu included (1) tutoring in individual or small-group sessions to teach concepts, assist with homework, and enhance study skills; (2) behavioral contracting for school performance to increase specific behaviors and decrease others, and to enhance motivation for homework completion and studying; (3) assistance in the school setting, to enhance youths' attention skills or provide individualized support in school; and (4) consultation with teachers to enhance tutoring effectiveness or behavioral management.

## Peer Relations

Given the central role of peer influence in the adolescent progression of CD, peer relations were an important focus of the adolescent prevention program. Associated action plans focused on individual meetings with youth, family meetings, and group meetings incorporating positive peers. Risk factors (listed below) emphasized affiliations with deviant peers and engaging in antisocial behavior (Dishion & Tipsord, 2011).

Conversely, friendships and affiliation with normative, nondeviant peers were evaluated as protective factors, given their links with productive time use and prosocial orientation (Fergusson, Lynskey, & Horwood, 1996). Indeed, research has shown that youth with early conduct problems who have fewer delinquent friends are more likely to decrease their conduct problem behaviors over time than those with more deviant friends (e.g., Lahey, Loeber, Burke, & Rathouz, 2002).

Triannual assessment risk factors in the peer domain included (1) current involvement with deviant peers, (2) an interest in activities engaged in by deviant peers (high-risk, antisocial activity), (3) a high level of exposure to deviant peer-group activities (e.g., exposure due to neighborhood or sibling influences), and (4) rejection or victimization by peers and hostile attitudes toward peers. Protective factors included (1) current involvement in positive peer-group activities, (2) interests and leisure-time pursuits that were prosocial and normative, and (3) high-quality friendships with nondeviant peers.

Prevention efforts to improve peer relations focused both on improving opportunities for exploring interests and developing skills in the context of positive peer interactions, and improving self-control and thoughtful decision making. Specific prevention strategies on the Fast Track menu included (1) individual or small-group meetings with youth to discuss problems and identify action plans, to provide support, to enhance skill development, and to provide opportunities for youth to discuss their feelings and current concerns; (2) behavioral contracting for social-behavioral growth, to increase specific behaviors and decrease others, and to enhance motivation for applying self-control and avoiding problem behaviors or potentially problematic situations; (3) mentoring, with Fast Track volunteer mentors or mentors provided by community agencies, to provide recreational opportunities, positive models for identity development, and increased supervision; and (4) supporting and facilitating youth participation in school or community groups to support positive peer affiliations and positive youth engagement in school and community (e.g., facilitating memberships and participation in school clubs, sports activities, church groups, hobby clubs, teen centers, or summer work programs.)

## Parenting and Adult Involvement

Parents continue to play a key role in the persistence or desistance of their children's conduct problems in adolescence. In particular, parent–youth communication, monitoring, and supervision become particularly important as adolescents attain more autonomy (Racz, McMahon, & Luthar, 2011; Stattin & Kerr, 2000). The Fast Track triannual assessments focused on these important aspects of the youths' relationships with parents and with other significant adults, tracking conflict as a risk factor, and close, supportive relationships characterized by open communication and trust as protective factors (Stattin & Kerr, 2000). Services linked with this area of focus included parent meetings and family meetings to foster productive parent–adolescent communication and conflict resolution, joint problem solving, and effective planning and monitoring. Especially in families in which attaining positive parental involvement was difficult, Fast Track also encouraged other positive adult–youth relationships, based on research indicating that positive and supportive relationships with adults outside the family (e.g., extended family member, coach, neighbor) can reduce risk for conduct problems (Estroff & Zimmer, 1994).

Risk factors assessed in the parenting and adult-involvement domain included (1) high levels of conflict with parents and/or other adults, including teachers or authority figures; (2) problems with acting out or defiant behaviors in school or neighborhood settings; (3) unsupervised time; and (4) current involvement in covert antisocial behaviors, such as substance use (including smoking) or sexual activity. Protective factors included (1) positive and involved relationships with parents or other adults, (2) positive family communication skills, (3) supervised leisure-time activities, and (4) high-quality monitoring provided by parents or other adults.

For all youth, Fast Track action plans included a role for parents. The specific goals that YCs had for parents varied across families. In some cases, YCs worked actively to promote parenting skills, including monitoring youth activities, communicating with youth, reducing family conflict, and developing behavioral contracts to manage problem behaviors. In other cases, where parental limitations or circumstances limited the potential for parental change, goals focused on maintaining parental support for services to be provided directly to the youth by Fast Track, the school, or community agencies. Prevention strategies included (1) problem-solving meetings with parents, focusing on monitoring, limit setting, and communication skills; (2) family problem-solving meetings, involving intensive efforts to improve parent–youth relationships and communication, reduce parent–youth conflict, and improve parental monitoring; (3) short-term crisis intervention, to help parents utilize effective problem-solving skills under stressful circumstances, such as a serious school problem (leading to school suspension), an atypical family problem (sibling crisis, marital breakup, death of family member), or a serious youth problem behavior in the community; and (4) referral to community service agencies for parents who experienced more chronic crises and required general support for living skills or personal or family

adjustment problems (including substance abuse, chronic domestic instability, or chronic economic crises).

## Identity Development

The fourth domain targeted by Fast Track focused on youths' attitudes,
values, and beliefs, with a particular focus on their emerging sense of
identity and self-efficacy. Beliefs supporting the acceptability of antisocial behavior, glorification of violence, and preference for high-risk
activities were identified as important risk factors (Henry et al., 2000).
Conversely, a positive sense of self, a strong ethnic identity, a sense of
control and self-efficacy, along with hope regarding the future served
as protective factors that contributed to efforts at education and vocational development, and reduced risk for antisocial activity (Luthar &
Zigler, 1991; Markus & Nurias, 1986). Associated action plans focused
on individual meetings with youth, group meetings with a vocational
focus, and the inclusion of adult mentors.

The triannual assessment focused on the following risk factors in
this domain: (1) lack of positive goals or future orientation, (2) attitudes
that glorified violence or other antisocial activities, (3) demonstration
of health-endangering behaviors, (4) the absence of conventional norms
and appropriate empathy/social concerns, and (5) impulsivity and poor
decision-making skills. Protective factors included (1) interpersonal relationships and environmental niches that provided models of conventional, prosocial norms and that supported the development of empathy
and social concern; (2) a positive sense of self and positive ethnic identity;
(3) a positive health orientation; (4) interests and motivation to support
the future development of vocational skills and career development; (5)
ability to make independent decisions; and (6) a future goal orientation.

Prevention strategies on the Fast Track menu that targeted a positive identity development included individual or small-group meetings
with youth to provide support for the development of personal future
goals and the acquisition of skills needed to pursue their interests and
goals. These meetings also allowed staff to facilitate youths' problem
solving and informed decision making about key life decisions that may
have affected their adaptation (e.g., coping with risky life circumstances;
coping with family dysfunction; and decisions about behavior, peers,
substances, and sexual activity). YCs could also recommend vocational
interest enrichment activities to facilitate youths' goal setting, motivation for school achievement, and goal attainment, and to enhance the
development of interests and skills for future vocational success. They
included individually tailored activities, such as the opportunity to complete a vocational inventory of job interests and feedback, interviews

with individuals in occupations of interest to youth, tours to observe work settings of interest to youth, and one to two sessions of "job shadowing" for an occupation chosen by the youth. The overall goals for these activities were to help youth (1) become engaged, interested, and ready for the development of vocational skills; (2) define what they wanted from life; and (3) see how they could achieve that goal. Vocational interest enrichment activities were often combined with youth meetings, as staff served as "coaches," preparing youth for the experience and then later debriefing the experience with youth. For example, before a job-shadowing activity, staff reviewed the responsibilities of a job observer or apprentice, covering issues such as dress, appropriate behaviors and attitude, and workplace expectations and rules. After the experience, staff discussed with youth their reactions and evaluations of the job and the workplace, helping youth clarify the characteristics of various job situations that did or did not appeal to them. In addition to these problem-solving and vocational interest workshops, staff offered special focus workshops, including workshops to support pride in black heritage and to help black youth prepare to deal with racial stigma.

## INTERVENTION PARTICIPATION RATES

After completing each triannual assessment, YCs selected from a menu to design an action plan for each youth. They then tracked youth and family participation in the recommended activities that included different combinations of family meetings, parent meetings, youth meetings, mentoring sessions, group meetings, academic support, and consultation.

In general, participation in the Fast Track intervention decreased modestly across years, primarily due to families moving out of the geographic area in which services could be provided. In a few cases, youth were unavailable due to custody changes or residential placement, or because of youth or parent refusal. Across the years of the adolescent phase of intervention, participant availability for intervention services decreased gradually, from 78% (grade 7) to 76% (grade 8) to 70% (grade 9) to 64% (grade 10). Levels of participation across the adolescent phase for the various intervention components are summarized in Table 6.2.

## PSYCHOMETRIC PROPERTIES OF THE TRIANNUAL ASSESSMENT

At the time when we developed and implemented the Fast Track adolescent phase, there were few guidelines available regarding the optimal

**TABLE 6.2. Participation in Adolescent-Phase Prevention Services**

| | Level of participation | |
| --- | --- | --- |
| Type of service | % participants receiving any | Median no. received (SD) |
| Parent meetings | 80% | 15.5 (16.3) |
| Youth meetings | 78% | 23.6 (24.5) |
| Formal family meetings[a] | 63% | 3.8 (5.8) |
| Group meetings | 73% | 6.4 (7.8) |
| Mentoring sessions | 31% | 3.1 (7.8) |
| Academic support | 64% | 34.2 (60.9) |
| Consultation[b] | 77% | 20.2 (26.5) |

[a]In addition to meetings with parents and youth, YCs sometimes organized formal problem-solving meetings that included the entire family.

[b]Consultation included school or agency contacts.

way to collect ongoing assessments for the purpose of tailoring intervention programming. We designed the triannual assessment in order to meet this need. Subsequently, we conducted some psychometric analyses to evaluate the reliability and predictability of this measure.

As noted earlier, when youth were in grades 6 and 7, the Fast Track staffing patterns changed, transforming from two intervention staff roles (EC, FC) to one intervention staff role (YC). In the first year that this transformation took place, the ECs and FCs were asked to complete the triannual assessment forms independently. This assessment allowed us to examine the interrater reliability of the measures, using data from the 73 subjects for whom interrater agreement information was available (for more information, see Schofield, 2009). Reliability varied across domains and was uniformly better for the ratings of risk factors relative to ratings of protective factors. Risk factors in the academic domain were most reliably rated (intraclass correlation coefficient [ICC] = .73), followed by risk factors in the adult involvement domain (ICC = .66), and peer relations domain (ICC = .65). Staff were less reliable in their ratings of risk factors associated with youth identity development (ICC = .51). In general, interrater reliability on protective factors was poor (ICC = .26 for academic achievement; ICC = .35 for peer relations; ICC = .10 for adult involvement, and ICC = .48 for identity development). These ratings were used to recommend levels and types of prevention support. Future prevention programming would benefit from additional research designed to improve the reliability of the assessments used to tailor pre-vention services to fit individual youth needs. Although it makes sense conceptually to focus on strengths (protective factors) as well as weak-nesses (risk factors), our findings suggest that a focus on risk factors might increase the reliability of intervention staff ratings.

We undertook additional analyses to determine whether these staff ratings improved the prediction of youth conduct problem development in ways that extended beyond standard research-based measures. For these analyses we examined growth in youth CD symptoms between sixth grade and ninth grade when we had administered structured diag-nostic interviews. We entered the following predictors in a regression equation to predict ninth-grade CD symptoms: family demographics, sixth-grade CD symptoms, and measures collected during the summer research interviews with each family in seventh and eighth grades. After these variables were accounted for, we then entered YC staff ratings of risk levels in seventh and eighth grades.

Taken together, family and child demographics (i.e., sex, race, site, family SES, baseline child behavior problems) predicted 12% of the variance in ninth-grade CD symptoms. When we added sixth-grade CD symptoms, they accounted for an additional 18% of the variance, and seventh- and eighth-grade risk factors (youth grade-point average, par-ent report of youth difficulties and risk factors, youth report of his or her difficulties and risk factors) accounted for an additional 7% of the variance in ninth-grade CD symptoms. However, even after accounting for demographics, earlier CD symptoms, and research-based measures entered, the YCs clinical ratings of risk and protective factors signifi-cantly improved the prediction of youth CD symptoms in ninth grade, contributing an additional 6% of the variance (see Schofield, 2009, for more details).

The finding that clinical ratings of youth risk and protective factors significantly improved the prediction of youth CD symptoms in ninth grade, above and beyond what could be predicted using a set of demo-graphic and youth risk factors, validates the use of clinical ratings to tailor prevention recommendations. YCs were able to rate early adoles-cents on a set of risk and protective factors with moderate reliability and predictive validity, in ways that out-performed standard research-based measures. Further research might reveal strategies to improve the reli-ability of these kinds of ratings, thereby further improving their predic-tive validity and clinical utility. These findings also provide some vali-dation of the four domains of functioning that our intervention model focused on during the early adolescent years to reduce risk for future conduct problems and antisocial behavior.

These analyses are in alignment with a substantial body of research that highlights the importance of risk and protective factors in better understanding progressions toward or away from problematic adolescent outcomes (e.g., Pollard et al., 1999; Stouthamer-Loeber, Loeber, Wei, Farrington, & Wikstrom, 2002). While the Fast Track model focused intensive intervention efforts during childhood, we hypothesized that later targeting of the four domains of intrapersonal and contextual factors would strengthen the intervention impact affecting trajectories toward antisocial behavior during early adolescence.

## CASE STUDIES

The two case studies provide an example of how individual families navigated the intervention services provided by Fast Track during the adolescent phase.

### Jeremiah and Grace Locke

During much of the adolescent phase, and because of new challenges in his relationship with his mother, Jeremiah showed moderate risk in adult supervision. The family conflict at home that had reemerged limited how much his mother monitored him, so Fast Track family and parent meetings focused on improving Grace and Jeremiah's communication. Jeremiah also showed moderate risk in peer relations and identity development: In seventh and eighth grades, he behaved impulsively in school and with friends. Identity development services were designed to help him be less impulsive, learn to make better decisions and, in the last 2 years of the intervention, develop vocational interests. Because he was cutting class with friends and talked about joining a gang when he was 14, his YC tried to expose him to more positive peers so he could form healthier friendships. The Fast Track services Jeremiah received varied over the 4 years. He received three times as many service contacts in the early adolescent years (90 during middle school) than in later years, based upon his risk levels assessed triennially. As Jeremiah entered high school, he began to show greater maturity and less impulsive decision making. He got an after-school job and spent less time with the friends involved in criminal activity. By 10th grade, during the last year of Fast Track services, Jeremiah was recommended for a low level of Fast Track services. He continued to receive contacts with his YC focused primarily on controlling his impulsive school behaviors and providing him with positive peer alternatives, as well as to address periodic family conflicts.

## Cindy, Susan, and Janice Steele

At the start of the adolescent phase of intervention, Cindy was assessed at high risk in the domains of academics, peer relations, and identity development. Since she had recently moved in with her aunt, Janice, Fast Track worked with the family to establish a positive daily schedule and to support adult supervision. Janice had a good relationship with Cindy and managed supervision well; hence, once a positive daily schedule was established, these Fast Track services shifted to periodic check-ins. Fast Track services concentrated on school challenges, working with teachers and school staff to put supports in place to help Cindy establish positive peer relations and reduce her risk of connecting with deviant peers, as well as to support her academic progress. An important shift in Cindy's situation as she got older was her own motivation to change. As a young adolescent, she was unhappy with herself and her situation. Her negative mood fueled impulsive behavior, but she was also open to talking with teachers and her YC about her difficulties. Academically, her goal was to maintain grades of Cs, which was challenging for her given her attention problems. Her YC worked with her at school, coordinating her efforts with Cindy's teachers and guidance counselor. Her YC also ran a weekly social club at school for Cindy to help her with friendships and connected with a mentor who saw Cindy weekly outside of the school context. These multiple Fast Track services were focused on improving her positive peer connections, helping her stay on-grade in school, and fostering a sense of positive identity and vocational interests. Cindy continued to receive a high level of Fast Track services through 10th grade. The total number of Fast Track service contacts varied from 70–100 per year across grades 7–10. When the Fast Track intervention ended, Cindy had shifted down to moderate risk levels in each area of academic, peer relations, and identity development.

# Chapter 7

# Outcomes during the Middle School and High School Years

This chapter presents the Fast Track intervention outcomes evident during the middle and high school years. In general, intervention-related gains faded during the middle school years, and then reemerged in later adolescence, when the Fast Track intervention led to reductions in antisocial behavior and fewer juvenile arrests. Mediation analyses documented a process in which the behavioral, social, and emotional gains made by Fast Track children in the elementary school years laid the foundation for these later-emerging effects on adolescents' antisocial behavior in the high school years. As will be evident in Chapter 8, major improvements in outcomes associated with the Fast Track intervention became even more apparent in the early adult years.

In the original plan for Fast Track, we hoped that intensive intervention during the early elementary years would significantly reduce youth risk for the escalation of CD and related risky behaviors (e.g., substance use, risky sexual activity) in adolescence. As noted in Chapter 5, Fast Track promoted early social-emotional competencies and interpersonal relationships in the targeted aggressive children. However, effects were relatively small in size, and a majority of the children still faced multiple adversities in their daily lives due to their family, neighborhood, and school disadvantage. When children transitioned from elementary school into middle or junior high school, they generally experienced reduced supports in the school context. That is, in the larger, more fluid secondary schools, youth were less likely to be closely monitored by teachers than they had been in elementary school, and they faced demands for more independent academic and behavioral functioning. In addition, as youth moved through puberty and transitioned into adolescence, normative changes occurred in their interpersonal relationships. They sought more independence from adults and spent more time socializing with peers. This shift increased their risk for involvement in deviant peer activity, substance use, and delinquency.

By early adolescence, there was a growing heterogeneity in the sample as some youth were more highly affected by these new risks than others. Due to variations in the timing of the middle school transition across different school districts, the characteristics of the secondary schools that youth attended, and the timing of puberty, risk exposure (and, conversely, protective supports) varied considerably for youth in the Fast Track study. Occasional rule-breaking and other antisocial behaviors were not uncommon, and a number of youth in the sample began to display more recurrent and serious early antisocial activity.

These variations in experienced school contexts and pace of individual social development affected the timing of youth risk and increased the challenges of predicting adjustment and detecting Fast Track intervention effects in early adolescence. In addition, as analyses began to focus more heavily on criminal outcomes during this period, we recognized that discrimination against minority youth may have affected risks in ways that were specific to the black youth in the sample. Corresponding site differences emerged in some of our primary outcomes during early adolescence, including how often youth of different races were arrested for engaging in similar conduct problem behaviors, and variation in the likelihood that youth of different races would initiate comorbid problems, such as substance use and risky sex during early adolescence.

## OUTCOMES DURING THE MIDDLE SCHOOL YEARS

In contrast to the positive intervention effects evident during the elementary school years, we found few differences between the intervention and control groups during the middle school years (CPPRG, 2010a). The pattern of effects observed in grades 6–8 is described below, focusing on the core domains of antisocial behaviors, social functioning, and academic progress.

### Antisocial Behavior

In the domain of antisocial behavior, the Fast Track intervention produced two effects in seventh grade: lower levels of hyperactivity behaviors (according to Parent Daily Report [PDR] ratings) and less self-reported delinquency. These were the only two main intervention effects that were significant out of a set of 16 rating scales collected during the middle school years. Outcomes in the antisocial domain with no significant intervention effects included: self-reported delinquency (eighth grade), PDR aggression (seventh and eighth grades), and externalizing behaviors on the Child Behavior Checklist (parent report in seventh grade; teacher report in sixth, seventh, and eighth grades). Given the few significant effects during these years, results must be interpreted cautiously.

In addition, we found reduced ADHD symptoms in structured diagnostic interviews (DISC; Shaffer, Fisher, Lucas, & Comer, 2003) for the subgroup of highest-risk youth in the sample. Given the goal of reducing CD and related psychopathology, Fast Track included structured diagnostic interviews with parents conducted every 3 years, starting when the children were in third grade. During this interview, they were asked to report on the set of symptoms that define CD and other disruptive behavior disorders (ODD, ADHD). Although rates of disorder were not reduced for the entire sample, consistent reductions emerged for youth at the highest risk (the top 3% on the screen score.) Initial intervention benefits were evident in third grade, and these continued through the middle school years, evident also at sixth and ninth grades (CPPRG, 2007). The first three time points in Figure 7.1 depict the levels of any externalizing symptoms for the highest-risk youth at grades 3, 6 and 9. At each time point, the highest-risk youth in the Fast Track intervention sample had significantly fewer symptoms of CD than the control condition. Across all three grades, the highest-risk Fast Track intervention children also had lower rates of ADHD symptoms. In third grade, they also had significantly lower rates of ODD symptoms and in ninth grade significantly

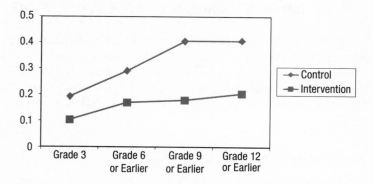

**FIGURE 7.1.** Cumulative rates of any externalizing diagnosis by either parent or child informant as a function of intervention among the highest-risk group.

lower rates of CD symptoms. The intervention effects on ODD and CD symptoms were not statistically significant in sixth grade, but there was a nonsignificant trend for lower CD symptom rates during that year.

Conceptually, the improvements in social functioning and self-control that Fast Track produced during the elementary years may have helped youth who were highly impulsive and disruptive develop a better capacity to inhibit their reactive and overactive behaviors. The Fast Track intervention focus on assisting parents to provide clearer consequences for problem behavior may also have helped the highest-risk youth acquire more accurate and adaptive expectations of consequences following disruptive behaviors, and this may have contributed to greater behavioral inhibition and reduced rates of overactive behaviors.

The intervention effect on reduced youth self-reported delinquent offenses in seventh grade was not seen on youth self-reported delinquency in sixth or eighth grades (CPPRG, 2007) and, as noted, the intervention effect on CD symptoms for the highest-risk group was in the right direction but not statistically significant in sixth grade. These findings suggest that Fast Track had some effects on reducing delinquency, perhaps associated with gains in inhibiting impulsive responding as evident in the hyperactivity finding, but the effects were variable over time.

## Social Functioning and Academic Performance

Fast Track promoted significant advantages in social skills and social competence during the elementary school years (CPPRG, 1999a, 1999b, 2002a, 2004); however, these benefits were not evident in middle school. Overall, youth from the intervention and control conditions demonstrated similar levels of social skills with peers and interpersonal relationships with teachers during the middle school years. Surprisingly, intervention youth reported higher levels of involvement with deviant friends in eighth grade than did youth in the control condition. It is possible that their improved social skills fostered more friendships—but with undesirable peers—during middle school. Increased involvement with deviant peers may then have contributed to a deterioration in their associations with other students and adults at their schools. However, it is important to note that this was an isolated finding that was not observed in any other year. Although Fast Track promoted academic benefits at school entry, when intensive reading tutoring was provided, evidence of academic benefits had faded completely by the end of elementary school (CPPRG, 2004).

Overall, the pattern of early elementary school intervention effects followed by reduced early adolescent effects is similar to the "fadeout" effects that have been reported with other kinds of early interventions with at-risk children, albeit those occurred after a shorter intervention, while ours was evident in the middle of a long 10-year intervention period. For example, a number of early childhood interventions for economically disadvantaged children that promoted early academic and behavioral improvements then documented fade-out of those benefits during the later school years (see meta-analysis by Protzko, 2015). At the same time, some of these programs produced longer-term benefits that emerged after the years in which intervention effects appeared dormant (Duncan, Ludwig, & Magnusson, 2007). For example, in the Perry Preschool Project intervention effects on intelligence scores disappeared by third grade, but lasting effects emerged later on important adult outcomes such as employment rates and criminal arrests (Duncan et al., 2007).

## OUTCOMES DURING THE HIGH SCHOOL YEARS

### Antisocial Behavior

*Arrests and Self-Reported Offenses*

Despite the sobering dearth of clear intervention effects during the middle school years, evidence supporting the long-term benefits of Fast Track emerged in later adolescence as data on antisocial behavior and crime accumulated through age 19 (CPPRG, 2010b). In order to capture both the frequency and the severity of criminal activity, official juvenile and adult arrest records were collected and scored. We created a lifetime severity-weighted index (Cernkovich & Giordano, 2001) to represent youth arrests. At each arrest, each offense was assigned a severity score ranging from 1 (least severe) to 5 (most severe). Severity level 1 involved status and traffic offenses. Severity level 2 included low-severity crimes such as breaking and entering, disorderly conduct, possession of controlled substances, shoplifting, vandalism, and public intoxication. Severity level 3 crimes reflected medium severity, such as simple assault, felonious breaking and entering, possession of controlled substances with intent to sell, and fire-setting. Severity level 4 contained crimes involving serious or potentially serious harm and included assault with weapons and first-degree burglary. Severity level 5 included all violent crimes such as murder, rape, kidnapping, and first-degree arson. We then summed the severity level of the most severe offense from each arrest from grades 6–12 (separately for adult and juvenile arrests).

By the end of high school, Fast Track intervention youth had significantly lower scores on juvenile crime as measured by the severity-weighted crime index derived from official juvenile court records.

Overall, the odds of being involved in court-recorded arrests was 29% less for intervention youth than for control youth. In addition, when we conducted additional analyses separately for crimes at different levels of severity, there was a significantly lower frequency for moderate-severity juvenile arrests; the rate for intervention youth was 24% less than for control youth.

Both court records and youth self-reports indicated intervention effects on the timing and onset of delinquent behavior. Specifically, Fast Track delayed the onset of juvenile court-record arrests; the odds of intervention youth *initiating* delinquency (based on juvenile arrests) was 77% of the initiation rate for control youth. Further, the intervention delayed the onset of the most severe forms of self-reported criminal behavior; the odds of high-risk intervention youths initiating self-reported delinquent behavior was only 82% of the initiation rate for control youth. These similar results across the two sources support the validity of these findings. Thus, intervention youth were less likely to initiate serious delinquent acts across this age period through the 12th grade, although no difference was observed for milder antisocial activity (e.g., fighting, theft).

Adult arrest records were also examined through age 19, revealing intervention effects on rates of severe arrests for the subgroup of highest-risk youth. However, the small numbers of adult arrests at this age limited our capacity to test sensitively for intervention effects at that point. Later analyses in young adulthood are presented in Chapter 8.*

The positive Fast Track impact on reducing the frequency of juvenile court-recorded arrests activity (as measured by the juvenile weighted-severity arrest index) and the delayed onset of serious delinquent behavior (evident in the court records and self-reports) is important and substantial. A few other early prevention programs have likewise promoted reductions in crime, including the Seattle Social Development Project impact on age 21 lifetime rates of court charges (Hawkins, Kosterman, Catalano, Hill, & Abbott, 2005) and the Linking the Interests of Families and Teachers program reductions in onset of police arrest (Eddy et al., 2003). Similarly, the Nurse–Family Partnership home visitation program had benefits for some participants, with the subset of children of unmarried, low-income mothers showing reduced arrests, convictions, and violations of probation (Olds et al., 1998). The Montreal Prevention Experiment (Boisjoli, Vitaro, Lacourse, Barker, & Tremblay,

---

* Adult crime through age 20 primarily consisted of youth who had committed adult criminal offenses in the few years between their exit from the juvenile court system and the age of 20. However, there were a relatively few exceptions involving juveniles who had been remanded to adult court while still juveniles.

2007), which included multiple child-focused and parent-focused prevention components like Fast Track, demonstrated a nonsignificant trend toward reduced arrest. However, Fast Track is one of the relatively few prevention studies to demonstrate significant preventive effects on youth arrests, and is the only prevention program targeted on high-risk children. The greater intensity and duration of Fast Track, relative to the Montreal Prevention Experiment, may have accounted for its strong effects on crime reduction.

### Externalizing Diagnoses

Parallel to effects seen at earlier ages and the data on reduced delinquency, Fast Track reduced disruptive behavior disorders as assessed by DISC interviews with parents and youth in 12th grade among the highest-risk group. In addition, Fast Track yielded cumulating effects on CD across the multiple years of implementation (CPPRG, 2011). This study was the first to demonstrate that a long-term prevention program can prevent psychiatrically diagnosed CD in the group of highest-risk children, with positive effects continuing for at least 2 years after intervention ceases (see Figure 7.1). Without intervention, only 18% of this very high-risk group remained free from any externalizing psychiatric disorder by age 18. With random assignment to intervention, this rate increased to 32%. This finding provides experimental evidence that is consistent with the developmental cascade model that posits the critical role of environmental factors in catalyzing antisocial development in early-starting children. As a result, more clinical and preventive resources should be offered to the highest-risk group of youth and their parents (Sherman, 2007).

Although the positive effects were sustained by grade 12 (i.e., 2 years after intervention ended), there was little evidence that the effect either grew or weakened during this period. This pattern is consistent with a cumulative dose model. That is, the magnitude of difference between the intervention and control groups was similar after grade 9 and grade 12. In general, few cases of disorder were identified in either group for the first time during high school, a finding that is consistent with theories of these disorders as generally starting earlier in life. To the extent that new cases are not initiated after age 15, one might speculate that preventive intervention does not need to continue past this age to prevent this particular outcome.

We conducted hazard analyses to assess whether new positive effects of intervention were found at each time point of measurement while the intervention was ongoing. That is, after the first 3 years of intervention, those children who had been randomly assigned to intervention were less likely to be diagnosed with CD, ODD, and ADHD than were control children. The second test discards those children who had already been diagnosed and examines those children who had not been diagnosed by third grade. Among this group, assignment to intervention had a positive effect, showing a lower rate of diagnoses between third and sixth grade, and among those children who had not been diagnosed by sixth grade, intervention again had a positive effect showing a lower rate of diagnoses between sixth and ninth grade. These findings buttress the rationale for long-term intervention with early-starting children. That is, as the intervention continued, new positive effects of intervention were found. When the intervention ceased, the positive effects were sustained but did not grow any larger. It should be noted that we did not employ the experimental manipulation that is necessary to rigorously test the rationale for sustained intervention. Such a test would have involved randomly assigning children to varying lengths of intervention. It is plausible that the positive effects of the intervention would have grown across adolescent development even if we had only provided 3 years of intervention in early elementary school. On the other hand, no other long-term follow-up studies of short-term intervention have yet yielded such growing effects. Future studies might examine these hypotheses experimentally.

## Health Service Outcomes

Conduct problems often lead to the need for costly professional services. For this reason, we tested for possible Fast Track intervention effects on the use of mental health and other health services in adolescence, through the end of high school (Jones et al., 2010). Because families typically seek treatment for CD symptoms through outpatient psychiatric services, outpatient pediatric/family practitioner services, or inpatient services, we assessed all of these outcomes.

Following grades 9–12, parents/primary caregivers and youth provided information on youths' use of health and mental health services in the past year. We assessed their reports of the number of the following services received by youth: pediatric health service visits; emergency department visits; general health service visits (including general hospital or emergency department); general health visits for youth emotional, behavioral, academic, drug, or alcohol problems; outpatient visits to a mental health professional for emotional or behavioral problems; and any inpatient mental health service. Analyses indicated that intervention youth had fewer general health service visits for any reason, fewer visits to pediatricians (including for emotional or behavioral problems), and fewer visits to emergency departments than control youth. By later adolescence (grades 11 and 12), intervention youth themselves also reported having fewer outpatient mental health service visits than did control youth. It was notable that the means for the intervention group were in the range of the means from our normative sample, indicating a beneficial prevention and normalization effect on professional health service utilization. Although we found significant differences between intervention and control groups in multiple service categories, model-derived effect sizes were relatively small, partly as a function of low base rates of services use at these ages. If group differences were to persist across years, however, the overall effect could grow cumulatively. Improvements in health status can eventually have an impact on other aspects of behavior and health in young adulthood. These findings are among the first to show that preventive intervention services for young at-risk children can lead to reductions in general health, pediatric, emergency department, and mental health services in adolescence.

## Other Aspects of Adolescent Functioning

In contrast to these indications of positive effects of Fast Track on aspects of adolescents' antisocial behavior during the high school years, the Fast Track intervention did not influence school outcomes, early sexual activity, and early substance use, although intervention effects on risky sexual behavior and substance use did emerge in young adulthood (see Chapter 8).

### School Outcomes

Although the developmental course of aggressive behavior correlates with the developmental course of school success, our findings (CPPRG, 2013) indicate that while the Fast Track intervention improved aggressive behavior, it did not improve long-term school success. By the end of first grade, the Fast Track intervention had successfully modified the key factors implicated in the negative cascade model of school maladjustment. That is, children in the intervention group had higher reading achievement scores and higher language arts grades, more positive social skills and peer relations, and reduced rates of aggressive-disruptive behavior at school than children in the control group. In addition, the intervention included the ongoing delivery of academic support services through 10th grade, albeit at reduced levels and only for children assessed with academic needs. Hence, it was disappointing to find that the early academic gains dissipated over time and failed to impact the longer-term school adjustment of the participating children. The dissipation of academic gains was evident quite early, as intervention effects on reading achievement were no longer significant at the end of third grade

(CPPRG, 2002a). It is unclear why the intervention was not more successful at changing academic outcomes, and how future prevention studies might be modified to strengthen their impact on academic outcomes.

One possible reason for the lack of impact on the later academic outcomes is that the kind of academic support that Fast Track provided was not effective, or alternatively, that it was provided at too low a dose or intensity to be effective. In the first year of academic tutoring (and until children mastered the skills), Fast Track used the evidence-based Wallach tutoring program (Wallach & Wallach, 1976). However, after children mastered that program, Fast Track focused tutoring on the areas of need suggested by classroom teachers. Often, this included an emphasis on helping with homework completion. Prior studies suggest that children with reading disabilities benefit most from intensive tutoring, utilizing well-informed and evidence-based programs that incorporate a systematic progression of skills and teaching techniques, led by certified teachers (Wasik & Slavin, 1993). The weekly or biweekly homework support by paraprofessionals that Fast Track provided may have been too little and too unfocused to remediate the core cognitive deficits undermining the school maladjustment of many of the high-risk youth.

In addition, as noted in Chapter 5, careful analyses of the Fast Track tutoring program in the early school years suggested that it was most effective for children who had reading skill delays without concurrent attention problems; the treatment effect size was much smaller for children with concurrent attention deficits (Rabiner et al., 2004). Improving the achievement of children with attention problems is a ubiquitous challenge, and the difficulty of doing so suggests that the Fast Track program may have been insufficient to meet the significant academic needs of the approximately 30% of the sample with clinically elevated attention deficits. Additional or alternative intervention approaches are likely needed to address the attention problems of this subgroup of aggressive children, focused on promoting their cognitive development and processing, although it is not yet clear which intervention approaches will work. Among children with ADHD, longitudinal studies have suggested that early and sustained medication may improve academic achievement (Scheffler et al., 2009), but rigorous, randomized trials have not documented positive medication effects on achievement (Molina et al., 2008, 2009), making it unclear whether medication could foster improvements in school success among aggressive children with severe, comorbid attention deficits. In recent years, a growing area of research has focused on early childhood interventions designed to foster the development of executive function skills (e.g., working memory, attention control) (for reviews, see Bierman & Torres, 2016; Diamond &

Lee, 2011). The goal of these early interventions is to promote growth in attention control during the developmental period when the prefrontal cortex is undergoing rapid growth. Clearly, these are areas of prevention research that are important to pursue, with a particular focus on their utility with children who have the combined problems of serious attention deficits and aggressive behavior.

One of the unfortunate consequences of many current school-based interventions designed to help students who enter school unprepared for the academic and social demands involves unintended and negative long-term effects. For example, Jimerson and Ferguson (2007) examined the impact of elementary school grade retention or placement in a "transition K–1" program to provide children with more time to mature and adjust to school demands. Controlling for initial levels of aggression, students who were recommended for the transition classroom, but were promoted, displayed lower aggression in eighth grade, compared to both groups of retained students. Their research and other studies suggest that grade retention can have short-term gains, but increases risk for aggressive behavior and high school dropout in later years. Similarly, our own causal modeling of the Fast Track data, using propensity score methods, suggests that placement in a self-contained classroom in the secondary school years increased the likelihood that youth would end school with a CD diagnosis (Powers, Bierman, & Coffman, 2016). The reasons for these adverse effects are not clear, but they may reflect peer contagion effects associated with placements that increase interactions with other high-risk aggressive youth or changes in teacher perceptions, expectations, and treatment once youth have been identified as in need of retention or other special education services (Dishion, Piehler, & Myers, 2008). It is possible that the positive early effects of Fast Track were undermined in later years, as the intervention may have inadvertently increased the visibility of the participating students' academic and behavioral deficiencies, leading to reduced academic expectations or biased attributions on the part of teachers and school personnel regarding their capacity to learn.

It is also possible that the timing of preventive interventions requires more careful consideration. Fast Track provided the most intensive set of services at school entry, based upon the hope that a good start in school would set children on a positive path that reduced the negative developmental cascade so often associated with aggressive behavior. Due to a concern about possible iatrogenic effects of group intervention at the transition into adolescence (Dishion et al., 1999), our model shifted to a primary reliance on individualized services during the middle school years. The current data suggest that the transition into middle school is a particularly challenging time for aggressive youth; in this high-risk sample, grades plummeted and rates of behavior disorder classification and self-contained placements doubled post-transition. So, although the intensive Fast Track prevention efforts at school entry produced a number of positive and significant effects, they did not buffer high-risk youth sufficiently from the challenges of the middle school experience and transition into adolescence (see also CPPRG, 2010b). Research is needed to identify effective preventive interventions that focus on aggressive youth during the preadolescent and early adolescent years as they prepare for and make this critical transition.

Finally, although Fast Track employed an adaptive intervention design in order to individualize the provision of academic intervention services, this aspect of the design was not highly structured. YCs met with classroom teachers to discuss students' needs for intervention. A more elaborate system for evaluating students' academic needs and linking them with evidence-based academic support components might have strengthened the intervention impact (Collins et al., 2004).

## Substance Use

Although most of the Fast Track effects on outcomes generalize across site, sex, and race, a more complex picture emerged for self-reported substance use rates from grade 4 through age 20 (i.e., 2 years post-high school). Race and geographical setting were examined by comparing intervention effects for rural white children, urban white children, and urban black children (there were no rural black children in our sampling across sites). In rural settings, the Fast Track intervention reduced the substance use of white youth, who smoked fewer cigarettes, drank less alcohol, did less binge drinking, and used less marijuana than youth in the control group (McMahon, Witkiewitz, & Wu, 2009). In contrast, when urban black children were considered, Fast Track intervention youth drank more alcohol and reported more binge drinking across time than did the control group.

## Sexual Activity

We found no evidence that Fast Track delayed the timing of sexual debut or significantly reduced pregnancy or STDs through age 17 (CPPRG, 2014). It is valuable to speculate about the possible reasons for the lack of significant intervention effects at this age period, although there were intervention effects on risky sexual behavior later in young adulthood (as described in Chapter 8). The expectation that Fast Track might reduce risky sexual activity was based upon our developmental model in which child aggression at school entry contributes to a negative cascade, fueling interpersonal conflict (with teachers, peers, and parents) and learning failures that undermine social control and school engagement. On the basis of this model, we anticipated that aggressive youth would often enter adolescence feeling alienated and disengaged from their peers and therefore vulnerable to the attractions of a deviant lifestyle that offered easy social affiliation and gratification (e.g., substance use, sexual activity) and allowed them to escape from restrictive (often punitive) school demands and behavioral controls (Capaldi, Crosby, & Stoolmiller, 1996; Schofield, Bierman, Heinrichs, Nix, & CPPRG, 2008). It was anticipated that promoting social competence and reducing aggression in elementary school might reduce risks in these other areas. However, Fast Track did not substantially change youth vulnerability to the attractions of early substance use and sexual activity during this adolescent age period and did not delay the timing of sexual or substance use debut. It may be that the early impact of Fast Track on improving social competencies and reducing aggression was not sufficiently strong to protect youth from opportunities for deviant peer affiliation in middle school, which provided them with a gateway to substance use and early sexual debut. Fast Track effects, while statistically significant, were small to moderate in size, and during adolescence did not move most youth into "normative" levels of aggressive behavior. Alternatively, the negative cascade model, while descriptive, may not be causal. That is, although early aggression may indicate risk for precocious substance use and sexual activity, additional factors may contribute to both aggression and the other outcomes. For example, theorists have also speculated that poor self-regulation and related deficits in key areas of neuropsychological functioning contribute both to overreactive aggressive responding and also to learning difficulties and impulsive decision making, including decisions regarding substance use and sexual activity (Crockett, Raffaelli, & Shen, 2006; Zimmer-Gembeck & Collins, 2003). In the present study, we found that kindergarten cognitive skills, including elevated inattention and lower levels of cognitive ability, significantly predicted the earlier initiation of sexual activity and adolescent pregnancy involvement for boys and girls. A critical question for future prevention design is the degree to which these early cognitive skills are malleable in psychosocial interventions and, if so, whether such improvements reduce risk for early and unprotected sexual activity during this age period.

One additional possibility is that the transition into middle school and its accompanying reduction in adult monitoring and increase in youth affiliation with deviant peers opened new opportunities and support for substance use and sexual activity that were not reduced effectively with the youth-focused case management that Fast Track provided during the middle school years. Interestingly, although certain child characteristics at kindergarten significantly predicted the timing of sexual debut and pregnancy (e.g., low cognitive abilities for boys, elevated inattention for girls), they were not associated with the timing of tobacco or alcohol/drug use initiation. The risks for substance use appear more heavily associated with peer-group norms and opportunities, and hence require attention to the peer context to reduce risk. Certainly, additional research examining the Fast Track intervention, as well as future research examining alternative intervention approaches, is critically needed to better understand causal pathways and mechanisms associated with effective prevention targeting the trimorbidity of antisocial behavior, substance use, and risky sexual activity among youth with early-starting conduct problems.

Given the present findings, an expanded and differentiated prevention model may be needed to address alternative risk/protective mechanisms and diverging developmental trajectories characterizing youth at different developmental periods in varying ecological contexts, particularly over the transition into middle school when the contextual supports and peer-group risks change dramatically. Given that Fast Track effects on risky sexual behavior do emerge later in young adulthood (as will be seen in Chapter 8), it does appear that the early benefits of Fast Track did have long-term effects, but surprisingly, they were not apparent during this adolescent age period when risky sexual behavior first emerges for some youth.

## MEDIATION OF INTERVENTION EFFECTS DURING THE MIDDLE AND HIGH SCHOOL PERIODS

We also conducted mediation analyses to better understand the mechanism of action between factors targeted by Fast Track in the early years (e.g., children's self-regulation and social-cognitive processing, parenting skills) and later reductions in antisocial behavior. Our findings from three studies are summarized below to describe links between early Fast Track effects and later outcomes in middle school, the beginning of high school, and then the period of transition from high school to young adulthood. Following from our conceptual model in Chapter 2, we focused on the early Fast Track intervention effects on parenting and social cognitions.

### Mediation via Improved Parenting

Although there were few main effects of intervention in the middle school years, we found that parenting behaviors, impacted by the Fast

Track intervention, did affect aspects of youths' behavior in these difficult years. Reductions in parental harsh discipline in the early elementary school years (grades 1–3) predicted reductions in CD symptoms in sixth grade (Pasalich, Witkiewitz, McMahon, Pinderhughes, & CPPRG, 2016). In addition, the intervention's promotion of early parental warmth in grades 1 and 2 predicted reductions in callous and unemotional traits in seventh grade. Thus, Fast Track improved parenting in ways that, in turn, improved two important youth outcomes.

## Mediation via Improved Social-Cognitive Skills

Intervention effects on social cognitions in elementary school also led to later reductions in youths' self-reported delinquency at the beginning of high school (ninth grade). Specifically, increasing benign interpretations of peer provocations, increasing competent social problem-solving skills, and decreasing the degree to which children expected positive outcomes for aggressive behavior in elementary school each contributed partially to reduced adolescent delinquency (see Figure 7.2; Dodge, Godwin, & CPPRG, 2013). These findings provide the most rigorous evidence to date testing how early social-cognitive processes influence subsequent adolescent problem behaviors.

Virtually all prior tests of a social-cognitive model of the development of adolescent antisocial behavior have been purely descriptive cross-sectional or prospective studies (Dodge, Coie, & Lynam, 2006). The current findings are more convincing, as they are based on an intervention experiment in which social-cognitive processes were altered through random assignment to intervention. When children improved these processes through intervention during elementary school, they decreased their antisocial behavior during adolescence. These social-cognitive processes are a major psychological mechanism through which life experiences are stored and represented internally to guide later behavior. The three crucial social-cognitive processes that emerged in the Fast Track findings (i.e., making benign rather than hostile attributions about others' intentions, generating competent responses to social challenges, and evaluating the unfavorable outcomes of aggression) are by no means the only social-cognitive processes that might be important, but both theory and empirical findings support their central role. These findings echo the importance of children's hostile attributions and outcome expectations in mediating the effect of a more limited cognitive-behavioral intervention at an earlier early adolescent age period (Lochman & Wells, 2002).

Many programs to prevent antisocial behavior in children follow a logic model that focuses on promoting children's social competence, particularly social-cognitive skills, as proximal targets designed to

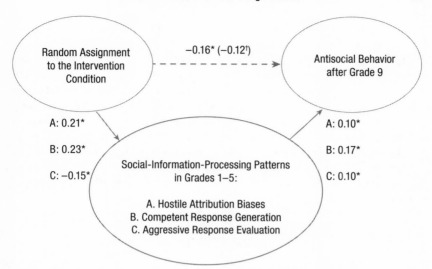

**FIGURE 7.2.** Structural equation model depicting the influence of random assignment to the intervention condition on antisocial behavior (assessed after children completed grade 9), as mediated by three social-cognitive processes. * indicates $p < .05$. † indicates $p < .10$. From Dodge, Godwin, and CPPRG (2013). Copyright © 2013 Association for Psychological Science. Reprinted by permission.

reduce distal problem behaviors. In our case, the logic model follows a developmental cascade approach (e.g., Dodge, Greenberg, Malone, & CPPRG, 2008). This logic model has not often been tested to determine how programs achieve their outcomes or to identify the important proximal indicators of success. These findings validate the logic model, demonstrating that improving these skills fostered positive long-term outcomes.

## Mediation via Improved Academic, Self-Regulation, and Interpersonal Skills

More recently, a broader test of the Fast Track logic, or developmental cascade, model was conducted by examining links between children's improvement in three different domains (academic, self-regulation, and interpersonal skills) measured during the elementary school years (ages 6–11) and later crime and delinquency (based on court records of juvenile and adult arrests and self-reported delinquency through age 20) (Sorensen, Dodge, & CPPRG, 2015). The three capability domains were measured as latent constructs using multiple measures we collected during the elementary school period. Mediation was assessed by a novel three-stage decomposition approach that had been pioneered by Heckman, Pinto, and Savelyev (2013). Our analyses indicated that improvements in children's self-regulation and social functioning during elementary school significantly predicted reduced risk for delinquency and crime outcomes through age 20, mediating the intervention impact on these outcomes. In contrast, intervention-produced improvements in proximal academic outcomes during the elementary years mediated intervention effects on adolescents' reduced use of mental health services. Thus, all three proximal skill domains served as active mechanisms fostering distal intervention effects, but they differentially affected different types of outcomes.

## CASE STUDIES

We turn now to how Jeremiah and Grace and Cindy and Susan were doing as a result of the adolescent-phase intervention.

### Jeremiah and Grace Locke

As Jeremiah started middle school, the family moved to a somewhat safer neighborhood. Jeremiah still observed occasional violence in the neighborhood and he sometimes was threatened, but overall the area was safer than their prior residence. Grace attained a full-time job, which eased some of their financial difficulties, and in general, she felt less stressed. During the early adolescent years, Jeremiah and Grace experienced an upturn in their conflict. Jeremiah wanted more freedom and autonomy and Grace reacted initially with negative discipline, eliciting noncompliance and disrespect from Jeremiah. Feeling tired of the ongoing conflict, Grace withdrew and pulled back in her supervision of Jeremiah. During these early adolescent years, Jeremiah also expressed more dissatisfaction with himself, including feeling bad about being black. However, as Jeremiah moved through adolescence, things improved for him and his family. By the time he turned 14, Grace was able to shift to more positive parenting, and parent–child conflict declined. Jeremiah reported more positive feelings about his race and himself, more generally. By age 15, Jeremiah had established positive connections in their new community; he was playing basketball at the YMCA and attending church. Grace told him that she was proud of him when he cleaned the house, stayed out of trouble in school, and stayed away from drugs. They talked a lot about finishing high school, whether with a diploma or general educational development (GED) certificate. Grace shared her difficult experiences in school and explained why she pursued her GED as an adult. Jeremiah felt that his mom supported him and he could talk with her about key pressures with peers and in school. As the Fast Track intervention ended, their parent–child relationship was positive and Jeremiah also felt connected to his teachers. He had set college as a goal.

## Cindy, Susan, and Janice Steele

During the early adolescent years, Cindy continued to live with her aunt. With Janice's support, in seventh and eighth grades, Cindy tried new activities—Girl Scouts and volleyball—which she really enjoyed. But she continued to struggle with depression, anxiety, and conflict with peers. Over time, with opportunities to form friendships with other teens through her new activities, Cindy began to feel more positively about herself. She also became quite interested in some of the vocational possibilities she learned about through Fast Track and set her sights on attending a vocational program after high school.

Although Susan's stress level rose and fell with job losses and financial problems, major family illness and death, she felt less stressed than in earlier years. She was able to stay positively connected with Cindy and support Janice's daily guardianship. With the transition to high school ahead of her, Cindy began spending more time at home with her mother and family. Unfortunately, this led to an escalation of mother–daughter conflict. In ninth grade, Susan and Cindy's fighting became physical and Cindy's emotional distress escalated. She was placed in a residential facility for a short stay. A brief time home was marked by more fighting and she returned to the facility. Cindy's residential treatment also led to a complete psychoeducational assessment that identified a learning disability. She began receiving special education services in ninth grade. Perhaps as a function of the intensive therapy and family work, and perhaps also as a function of these increased services at school, Cindy's behavior and grades improved.

As Fast Track was ending in 10th grade, Cindy had returned home to live with her mother and family. With the transition into high school, her special education services had been discontinued. In the next few years, her school attendance became more sporadic and she began drinking and smoking marijuana. She was picked up by police for underage drinking and disorderly conduct. Despite the significant investment of Fast Track services and positive accomplishments Cindy and her family made during the intervention years, her situation was unstable at the end of Fast Track. It was unclear whether she would finish school and whether she would overcome her substance abuse problems or they would undermine her future.

## SUMMARY

Despite the lack of clear intervention effects during the middle school years, clear effects of Fast Track on various externalizing behaviors emerged during the high school years. As illustrated in the case study examples, the youth and families served by Fast Track often faced multiple adversities, and substantial variation in youth adjustment was evident by the late adolescent years. Overall, however, despite the challenging life circumstances of the youth and families, Fast Track had a positive impact on its targeted goals. Relative to youth in the control group, youth in the Fast Track intervention group had lower rates of juvenile arrests and later onset for self-reported delinquent behaviors. Among the children who had the highest screen scores in kindergarten, the Fast Track intervention substantially reduced their rate of externalizing diagnoses. However, the Fast Track intervention did not have effects on academic outcomes, substance abuse, or risky sexual behavior during early and mid-adolescence. Our mediation analyses revealed that increases in parent warmth, decreases in harsh punishment from parents, and increases in child social-cognitive skills during the elementary school years accounted (at least partially) for reduced conduct problems and reduced callous-unemotional behaviors in early adolescence. More broadly, intervention-related growth in self-regulation and social competence during the elementary school years partially mediated intervention effects that led to a reduction of arrests in late adolescence, whereas intervention improvements in academic skills mediated intervention effects that led to a reduction in mental health service needs.

# Chapter 8

# Major Prevention Outcomes

This chapter focuses on the early adult outcomes of Fast Track, including the serious antisocial behavior that Fast Track was ultimately designed to prevent. In the elementary, middle, and high school years leading up to early adulthood, gains on intermediate outcomes were promising. As summarized in Table 8.1 (and reviewed in more detail in Chapters 5 and 7), children in the Fast Track intervention group showed improved social and academic functioning and reduced conduct problems in elementary school.

For children with the highest risk levels of early aggression in the sample, the intervention significantly reduced levels of disruptive behavior disorder symptoms starting in third grade through the end of high school. Although few intervention effects were evident during the middle school years, by high school, adolescent arrests were less frequent and less severe among youth in the Fast Track intervention compared to the control group.

Now we turn to the ultimate question: Was the Fast Track program successful in reducing the serious antisocial outcomes for the aggressive children who screened into the program 20 years earlier? Because of the length of time between screening and outcome, this question represents a particularly strict test of the prevention hypothesis. In this chapter, we describe important findings from analyses conducted when the sample transitioned into young adulthood as assessed at age 25. We also explore Fast Track intervention influences on typologies of offending behaviors from kindergarten through early adulthood. In addition, we review several analyses that explore the biological underpinnings of risk for CD,

**TABLE 8.1.  Summary of Fast Track Effects on Primary Participant Outcomes**

| | Elementary school | Middle school | High school | Young adulthood |
|---|---|---|---|---|
| Externalizing behavior—school and home | Grade 1–5: *Positive effects* | Grade 6–8: *No effects* | *No effects* | *Positive effects* |
| Psychopathology (CD, ODD, ADHD symptoms) | Grade 3: *Positive effects for highest risk* | Grade 6: *Positive effects for highest risk* | Grades 9 and 12: *Positive effects for highest risk* | *Positive effects* |
| Crime and delinquency | Not assessed | Grade 7: *Positive effects* <br> Grade 8: *No effects* | Grades 9–12: *Positive effects* | Age 25: *Positive effects* |
| Risky sexual behavior | Not assessed | Not assessed | *No effects* | Age 25: *Positive effects* |
| Academic outcomes | Grade 1–3: *Positive effects* <br> Grade 4–5: *No effects* | *No effects* | Grades 9–12: *No effects* | Age 25: *No effects* |
| Social competence and peer relations | Grades 1–5: *Positive effects* | Grade 7: *No effects* <br> Grade 8: *Negative effect* | Not assessed | Not assessed |

*Note.* Based on the Fast Track intervention research described in Chapters 5, 7, and 8. The table summarizes the results of published Fast Track outcome studies.

and the action of biological markers as mediators and moderators of adult antisocial outcomes. As you will see, as Fast Track participants moved into their young adult years, very clear positive intervention effects emerged on multiple important life outcomes.

## MAJOR LIFE OUTCOMES IN EARLY ADULTHOOD

Although a number of prior intervention studies have reduced children's antisocial behavior in the short-term, no prior program has followed kindergarten-age early-starting aggressive children into adulthood to evaluate long-term benefits. To assess the effect of Fast Track on young adult outcomes, we assessed participants at age 25, 19 years after they started the program and a full 8 years after intervention activities ended (Dodge et al., 2015). Administrative record reviews were collected, and psychiatric interviews were conducted with participants. Peers were also interviewed to provide independent perspectives on participant adjustment unbiased by program participation. Court records were collected at the local sites and were supplemented using a national database that included all adult arrests, adjudications, and diversions, with data available for 92% of the sample. The sample became increasingly dispersed in the adult years, making home interviews very difficult to collect, and hence adult measures often involved phone or Internet-based interviews.

## Court Records of Criminal Arrest

Adult criminal records were coded to reflect the severity and frequency of crimes committed up to age 25. Frequency was multiplied by severity across all lifetime convictions to create an overall severity-of-crime index. Violent crimes were coded at severity levels 1–3. Severity 1 included crimes such as driving under the influence (DUI) and carrying a concealed weapon; severity 2 crimes included robbery and first-degree burglary; and severity 3 included aggravated/armed robbery, murder, rape, kidnapping, sex offenses, and first-degree assault. Crimes involving illegal drugs were coded as severity levels 1 and 2; severity 1 included possession of illegal drugs, whereas severity 2 included manufacturing and possession with intent to sell. Severity levels for the property and public order crimes category ranged from 1–3.

Severity by frequency indices were analyzed for conviction data through age 25 for each of these three types of crime. Analyses revealed a significant reduction in violent crime associated with Fast Track intervention across the four sites, with the intervention showing a 31% reduction in violent crime relative to the control group (Dodge et al., 2015). Fast Track intervention also produced a 35% reduction in crimes involving illegal drugs across the four sites. No effects emerged on property and public order crimes. The reduced levels of adult criminality (violent and drug crimes) represent an extension of the intervention benefits that emerged during the high school years, when the Fast Track intervention group had lower rates of juvenile arrests than the control group (CPPRG, 2010b). These findings indicate a dramatic reduction in convicted crimes rates resulting from the Fast Track violence prevention program. These results provide the essential justification for the Fast Track project because they demonstrate that it is possible to reduce by 31% the number of violent and drug-related crimes committed by aggressive young children at risk for developing a lifetime pattern of chronic criminal behavior.

## Mental Health and Adjustment

Fast Track interviewers, who were unaware of the intervention versus control group status of the young adults, asked participants questions about eight domains of adult functioning: externalizing psychopathology, internalizing psychopathology, substance abuse, criminal conviction, risky sexual behavior, aggression toward partners and offspring, education and employment, and general well-being. Each participant was also invited to nominate a peer for an independent interview about the participant targeting the same domains of functioning.

Analyses of these interview responses revealed that Fast Track was effective in preventing costly adult psychopathology (Dodge et al., 2015; see Figure 8.1). Nineteen years after identification and 8 years after the intervention ended, individuals randomly assigned to the Fast Track intervention, compared to controls, displayed lower prevalence of externalizing problems (including reduced rates of antisocial personality disorder), internalizing problems (including reduced rates of avoidant personality disorder), substance use problems, and risky sexual behavior (see Figure 8.2). These findings were robust across both participant and

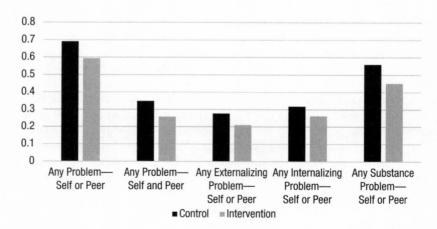

**FIGURE 8.1.** Rates of clinical problems at age 25 for intervention and control groups. From Dodge et al. (2015). Copyright © 2015 American Psychiatric Association. Reprinted by permission.

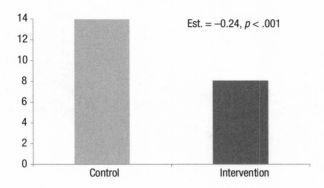

**FIGURE 8.2.** Intervention effects on risky sexual behavior at age 25.

peer raters. It is notable that, during the high school years, intervention benefits were largely evident in the domains of reduced antisocial behavior and reduced juvenile crime. A much broader pattern of benefits emerged in early adulthood, including intervention reductions in both substance use and risky sexual activity that became significant by age 25, as well as enhanced mental health.

Fast Track's efficacy did not differ across diverse subgroups of participants. That is, 12 "mini-replications" indicated that intervention effects were in the same direction for each of the four sites and three cohorts, and for males, females, blacks, whites, moderate-risk children, and high-risk children. Overall, the children who were screened for high levels of aggression in kindergarten and who received the Fast Track intervention had significantly fewer mental health and adjustment problems than similar children who did not receive Fast Track.

In addition to these long-term intervention effects, additional analyses suggest broad intervention benefits in other areas. Intervention participants reported experiencing higher levels of well-being and happiness (see Figure 8.3), and spanking their own children less often. In addition, the young adults who received the Fast Track intervention were significantly more likely than the control group to be civically engaged: They were more likely to register to vote and to actually vote (Holbein, 2017). Thus, intervention participants were more positively engaged in society than their counterparts in the control group, demonstrating positive citizenship and participation in democratic actions that create policy, rules, and resources for their community and larger society.

However, despite this broad set of positive outcomes, Fast Track did not have a significant impact on education or employment. Thus, the

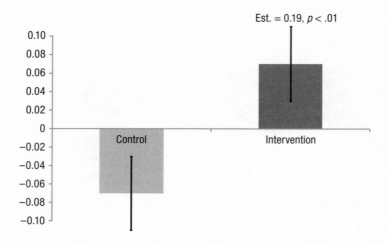

**FIGURE 8.3.** Intervention effects on young adult well-being at age 25.

program appeared to have stronger effects on assisting participants in areas of impulse control and the inhibition of risky, harmful, and illegal behaviors than it did on the set of skills and attitudes associated with improved educational outcomes and employment, at least at this point in young adulthood. It will be interesting to see if the program has any late-emerging effects on employment as the participants move further into adulthood; however, given the lack of intervention impact on educational attainment, employment benefits may not emerge.

These analyses contribute experimental evidence that a psychosocial intervention that promotes the social-emotional skills of high-risk aggressive children and targets improvements in their family interactions and peer-group experiences produces improvements in adult mental and behavioral health and reduces antisocial and criminal activity. The findings are consistent with a developmental cascade model in which changes in skills and social experiences early in life cascade into broader benefits many years later. The most important conclusion from this study to date is that a comprehensive, multicomponent, developmental science-based intervention targeted toward early-starting aggressive children can significantly reduce future violent crime and various forms of adult psychopathology. These findings should encourage policies and programs that acknowledge both the risk and the malleability of early-starting conduct problems and increase investment in early and multiyear prevention programming.

## PERSON-ORIENTED ANALYSES:
## TYPOLOGIES FOR ADULT CRIMINAL CONVICTIONS

Fast Track was designed based upon a developmental model of early-starting conduct problems. Hence, in addition to understanding intervention effects on adult outcomes, we were also interested in exploring Fast Track effects on developmental typologies of antisocial behavior. Accordingly, analyses were undertaken to identify the various developmental pathways to criminal convictions that emerged in the Fast Track sample through age 24 and to evaluate how those typologies were affected by the intervention. These analyses focused on criminal convictions for all officially recorded offenses. Because of the higher rates of convictions among males, these analyses focused only on males.

To develop typologies to adult convictions, we followed the strategy used by Jennings, Rocque, Fox, Piquero, and Farrington (2016), who followed men from age 8 to age 18 in the Cambridge Study in Delinquent Development. Jennings and colleagues constructed four groups of adults: *abstainers* (no convictions through age 18), *recoveries* (those who were convicted of crimes in early childhood but who had fewer than two convictions in ages 13–18), *life course persistent* (those who had criminal convictions in childhood and at least two convictions through adolescence, ages 13–18), and *adolescent limited* (no childhood convictions, but had convictions in adolescence). These four groups had significantly different adult adjustment.

To identify similar typologies in the Fast Track sample, the criminal convictions of boys in the sample were inspected during three developmental periods: childhood (age 13 and younger), adolescence (approximately ages 14–18), and post–high school through young adulthood (approximately ages 19–24). Focusing on convictions during the post–high school years allowed us to examine ongoing persistence of criminal behavior as the boys in the program moved into young adulthood. Four groups of youth were constructed (Goulter, Godwin, & CPPRG, 2018). *Abstainers* were those youth with no convictions over the entire time frame (ages 6–24); 39% of intervention youth and 33% of control youth fell into this category. The *adolescent limited* group (convictions during ages 6–18, but no convictions during ages 19–24) included 14% of the intervention youth and 11% of the control group youth. The *adult starters* (no convictions prior to age 19, but one or more convictions in ages 19–24) comprised 16% of the intervention and 18% of the control samples. The *life course persistent* group was defined as those with at least one conviction in each of the later time periods (ages 14–18 and ages 19–24) regardless of convictions prior to age 14; this group involved

32% of the intervention group and 38% of the control group. Interestingly, the rate of men from the intervention group in the life course persistent group was nearly the same as the rate of men in the normative sample (31%), suggesting that intervention had moved the at-risk youth into the normative sample range of offending.

Intervention effects on typology placement were examined with full-information maximum likelihood multinomial logit models controlling for intervention, site, cohort, race, and initial screen score. Each of the three offending groups of participants (other than the abstainers) was compared to the abstainers group. Intervention decreased the probability of being in the life course persistent group relative to the abstainers group (odds ratio [OR] = 0.62, $p$ = .04). These analyses indicate that the significant Fast Track intervention effects on males' criminal convictions was due primarily to the diversion of about 6% of the males from the life course persistent group, representing a 16% reduction in the number of individuals exhibiting a life course persistent trajectory. It was only by the late adolescent and young adulthood periods that conviction data reflected the dramatic intervention effects reported here for the entire intervention sample, and not just the highest-risk males of the intervention group, as was indicated by the late adolescent crime data. Some boys who might have been life course persistent instead became adolescence limited or abstainers. The fact that there was a 31% reduction in violent offending by age 25 suggests that there was an overall reduction of these offences in most of the intervention group, especially among intervention males who would otherwise have been part of the most problematic persistent trajectory group.

## MODERATION AND MEDIATION OF FAST TRACK EFFECTS ON YOUNG ADULT OUTCOMES

Fast Track was a psychosocial intervention, designed to promote positive supports and protective factors in the home and school socializing environments of high-risk youth, and designed to boost the social, social-cognitive, and self-control skills of participating children. Prior research has suggested that certain genetic factors may increase youth risk for developing early aggression and later antisocial behavior. It was of interest to understand how the psychosocial Fast Track intervention may have affected youth who varied on genetic risk factors, and whether genetic risk influenced intervention outcomes.

These analyses focused on the gene encoding of the glucocorticoid receptor (NR3C1). Glucocorticoid receptors influence the way that the hypothalamic–pituitary–adrenal (HPA) axis responds to environmental challenges and stress. Boyce and Ellis (2005), among others, have suggested that *NR3C1* genotypes represent an index of "biological sensitivity to context." Children with higher sensitivity to context are thought to be more responsive to variations in the quality of the socializing influences that affect them, whereas children with lower sensitivity to context are less affected by their socializing contexts. Children with higher sensitivity may flourish under conditions of high socialization supports, but show amplified negative developmental outcomes when exposed to socialization adversity (Boyce & Ellis, 2005). In a parallel fashion, theorists have speculated that children with high sensitivity to context may be more responsive to interventions that improve socialization contexts than children with lower sensitivity to context.

One study (Albert, Belsky, Crowley, Latendresse, et al., 2015) tested a gene × intervention hypothesis in the Fast Track sample by examining intervention response on any externalizing psychopathology at age 25 among children who varied on the glucocorticoid receptor gene *NR3C1*. Due to concerns regarding population stratification and genetic analyses, black participants were excluded from the analyses. They found that, among white children, a variant of *NR3C1* identified by the single-nucleotide polymorphism *rs10482672* (A allele) was associated with increased risk for externalizing psychopathology in the control group and decreased risk for externalizing psychopathology in the intervention group. In other words, in the control group, children with that particular genetic variant were more harmed than other children in the sample by exposure to adverse socialization supports, making them more likely to develop externalizing psychopathology without intervention. In contrast, in the intervention group, children with that genetic variant benefited more than other children from the Fast Track intervention supports, making them less likely to develop externalizing psychopathology with intervention. Specifically, among white children who were carriers of the A allele, 18% of treated children as compared to 75% of control children manifested any externalizing psychopathology at age 25 follow-up. This finding is important not just because it suggests a genetic moderator of the intervention, but because it suggests that a certain active mechanism (biologically based sensitivity to stressors) could be influenced by intervention.

A second study tested for gene × intervention interactions at different developmental periods that might mediate the longer-term intervention effects on young adult outcomes (Albert, Belsky, Crowley, Bates, et al., 2015). Their analyses followed three steps. First, they tested for genetic main effects on pretreatment risk variables. Children who carried the A allele showed several elevated risks at baseline, before the intervention began, with elevated levels of anxious-depressed and thought-problem symptoms relative to other children in the sample. This finding is consistent with prior research in which glucocorticoid signaling was found to be related to internalizing psychopathology. The second step of the analyses involved testing gene × intervention effects on the proximal developmental phenotypes during childhood and adolescence. The externalizing disorder phenotype was defined by ODD, CD, and ADHD symptoms assessed at grades 3 and 6, and by delinquency and substance use reported from grade 7 through age 20. Gene × intervention analyses documented that children with the high-sensitivity A allele were at increased risk for externalizing psychopathology in childhood and in adolescence if the children were in the control group, and that the reverse was true for children in the Fast Track intervention group. The third step was to test whether the proximal developmental phenotypes predicted the gene × intervention effect on young adult externalizing psychopathology outcomes. In this last step, the gene × intervention effects on child and adolescent psychopathology were found to mediate over half of the total gene × intervention effect on age 25 externalizing disorders. Interestingly, a portion of the total gene × intervention effect was accounted for by earlier effects in childhood, but 40% of the predictive effect emerged during the adolescent years when the full 10-year intervention was completed.

These latter results provide evidence that, for some white children, risk for adult violence and other externalizing problems is linked with genetic risk. However, they also indicate that interventions that improve child competencies and increase family and environmental supports can have a significant impact on children who possess those genetic risk factors. The fact that a genetic factor has been identified for white children but not black children does not mean that no genetic factor exists for black children, but it might suggest that contextual factors may be more important for the latter group. This does not mean, of course, that physiological processes are not at work in risk for violent behavior for children who do not have clear genetic risk.

A smaller study of such potential physiological processes was conducted at one of the sites (Durham) that was predominantly black. Carre, Iselin, Welker, Hariri, and Dodge (2014) examined whether the intervention effect on young adult males' reactive aggression at age 26 on a laboratory task, the Point Subtraction Aggression Paradigm (PSAP), was mediated by intervention effects on participants' hypothalamic–pituitary–gonadal (HPG) axis. The end product of the HPG axis is testosterone, and it was expected that testosterone differences on this type of task between young men in the intervention versus control conditions might account for differences in reactive aggressive behavior. Their results indicated that men who had received the Fast Track intervention had reduced aggression and reduced testosterone reactivity during the task, and that the reduced testosterone reactivity mediated the intervention effect on these men's aggressive behavior on the task. These findings suggest that the Fast Track intervention produced persistent changes in physiological processes that affected social-cognitive processes involving the way participants encoded, interpreted, and processed information about potential social threats and provocations in their environments. These effects of heightened testosterone reactivity in control adults may have been due to changes in amygdala reactivity to angry social cues. This is just one example of the importance of assessing neurobiological changes in response to early comprehensive interventions such as Fast Track.

## SUMMARY

The Fast Track intervention produced long-term reductions in the frequency and severity of violent crimes and drug-related crimes, evident at age 25. In addition, Fast Track effectively reduced externalizing problems (including antisocial personality disorder), internalizing problems, substance use problems, and risky sexual behavior in early adulthood and improved participant's feelings of well-being and happiness.

Similarly to the connection between adolescent and adult criminality, prior Fast Track effects on externalizing forms of psychopathology limited to highest-risk youth (at baseline screening) remained evident in early adulthood. In addition, benefits in adulthood (age 25) extended both to externalizing and internalizing diagnoses, and most notably, were evident across the full range of Fast Track children, not just the highest-risk youth.

In addition, these long-term effects on adult criminality (violent and drug crimes) represented an extension of the pattern of findings that we had observed in the high school years, when Fast Track youth had lower rates of juvenile arrests than did the control children. Thus, the intervention effect on this trajectory of serious outcomes was initiated in the prior developmental period of adolescence, and was maintained into the young adult years.

The overriding conclusion to be drawn from this latest Fast Track outcome data is that prevention of violent offending and serious substance use can be achieved, and that prevention does work when the multiple factors that contribute to such crimes are addressed in a meaningful way!

## Chapter 9

# Implications for Developmental Theory and Research on the Prevention of Violence

In 1993, Coie and colleagues described prevention science as a new research discipline being formed at the interface of diverse disciplines, including psychology, criminology, psychiatric epidemiology, human development, and education (Coie et al., 1993). Prevention science uses research on etiological risk/protective factors and developmental processes to inform intervention design, and then evaluates implementation processes and impacts using rigorous methodology. The overall goal is the promotion of societal well-being. In their seminal paper, Coie and colleagues suggested four principles for preventive interventions, noting that they should (1) address fundamental causal processes; (2) tackle risk factors before they become stabilized; (3) target those children who are at high risk for negative outcomes; and, when relevant, (4) include coordinated activities across multiple domains.

Each of these key principles informed the Fast Track design. We began with a carefully articulated developmental model that identified a set of cascading risk factors and processes that contributed to the escalation of behavior problems and emergence of antisocial activities over the long developmental period from school entry until the end of high school. This "consensus" developmental model (presented in Chapter 1) from the 1980s informed the design of the multicomponent Fast Track intervention model. The model targeted fundamental causal processes (parenting, child skills, classroom supports, peer relations) that mediated the relation between early risk factors and later antisocial outcomes. Intervention started early, at school entry, to address risk factors before they stabilized and to build protective competencies that could improve developmental trajectories.

In addition, taking an ecological perspective, we combined an indicated preventive intervention for high-risk children with a universal intervention intended to improve the classroom and school ecology to support all children in the intervention schools. Finally, because our developmental model identified cascading risk factors for antisocial outcomes across school and home settings and across social-emotional and academic domains, Fast Track included coordinated activities that changed over the developmental course from early elementary school through the transition into high school.

From the start, Fast Track was viewed as an opportunity to pull together what had been learned from numerous longitudinal investigations of the development of conduct problems and combine this with the best available intervention approaches to address the identified set of risk and protective factors. As a test of the consensus model of development of conduct problems, as well as a test of best practices, it was seen by us as a jumping off point for future efforts that would benefit from the data collected and both the mistakes and successes that those data revealed.

In the time since we began Fast Track in 1990 substantial advances have occurred in the scientific understanding of the development of children who are aggressive and in approaches to prevention and treatment. Advances in the methods and models used to study molecular genetics and developmental neuroscience are particularly noteworthy for their contributions to this field, as are recent developments in statistical methodology and interdisciplinary social science. In this chapter, we take a larger perspective on the Fast Track experiment, considering what we learned from this experience, new perspectives on the prevention of CD, and how our findings suggest next steps for the understanding and prevention of aggression and violence in children and youth.

## EVIDENCE SUPPORTING THE FAST TRACK MODEL OF THE PROGRESSION TO ADOLESCENT VIOLENCE

A key hypothesis guiding the Fast Track design was that children at high risk for future CD and antisocial outcomes could be identified at school entry on the basis of their elevated rates of early conduct problem behavior. This hypothesis was supported by longitudinal data; Table 9.1 shows the differences between the adult outcomes of the high-risk control group and the normative sample of children selected from the same schools. The findings at age 25 show that children who entered school

**TABLE 9.1. Percentage of Problematic Outcomes at Age 25 for the Fast Track Control Group and Normative Samples Drawn from the Same Schools**

| Problematic outcomes | Control (%) | Normative (%) |
|---|---|---|
| Any externalizing psychiatric disorder | 63 | 51 |
| Any substance use disorder | 53 | 46 |
| Antisocial personality disorder | 24 | 12 |
| Attention-deficit/hyperactivity disorder | 15 | 8 |
| Binge-drinking problem | 30 | 25 |
| Marijuana abuse | 10 | 9 |
| Serious substance use | 17 | 13 |
| Alcohol abuse disorder | 36 | 31 |
| Drug dependence disorder | 14 | 10 |

with high rates of conduct problem behavior developed much higher rates of substance abuse and mental health problems than their normative peers.

The Fast Track developmental model further hypothesized a negative developmental cascade, in which early risks increase exposure to later risks that, in turn, amplify the likelihood of adolescent violence and maladjustment. Specifically, we anticipated that families living in disadvantaged circumstances and unsafe neighborhoods often experience multiple adversities (chronic stress, lack of resources, family instability) that contribute to harsh and inconsistent parental discipline practices. In turn, exposure to harsh and inconsistent parental discipline, along with a lack of early sensitive-responsive support, can impede the development of the child social and cognitive skills that support school readiness. In particular, delayed language development, reduced emotional understanding, hostile attributional biases, and poor social problem-solving skills were anticipated, accompanied by poor impulse control and elevated conduct problem behaviors at school entry. These early academic and social-emotional deficits predict the child's display of externalizing conduct problems at school entry, which becomes the path leading toward later adverse outcomes.

Children showing this early-starting conduct problems profile and associated skill deficits at school entry are likely to alienate peers and struggle academically (Moffitt, 1993), fueling disengagement from school and alienation from the mainstream peer group and increasing the likelihood of rule breaking and rebellious behavior as they moved toward adolescence. Although these behaviors call for increased monitoring, supervision, and communication with parents, aggressive and rebellious youth are particularly challenging to parent. Without support, we anticipated that discouraged parents would frequently give up on their attempts to supervise their teenage youth, thereby increasing youth exposure to deviant peers and opportunities for antisocial activity.

Using the Fast Track normative and control samples, we tested this cascade model as shown in Figure 9.1 (Dodge, Greenberg, et al., 2008). Each of the seven predictor domains (early adverse context, harsh and inconsistent discipline, school social and cognitive readiness, early externalizing behavior problems, school social and cognitive failure, parental monitoring and communication, and deviant-peer associations) was significantly related to adolescent violence. This pattern held true for both boys and girls.

These findings reveal the complexity of the developmental processes that contribute to antisocial outcomes. First, multiple factors in diverse domains predict antisocial outcomes. Second, these risk factors are interrelated and develop in interdependent ways, as risks at earlier

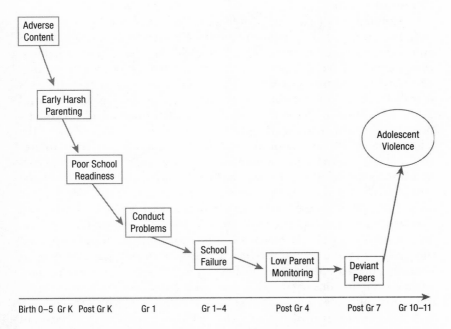

**FIGURE 9.1.** Hypothesized dynamic cascade model of the development of violent behavior.

time points increase vulnerability to subsequent risks across the course of development from early childhood through adolescence. Third, accumulating risks each play unique and incremental roles in predicting later antisocial outcomes. This patterned sequencing across phases of development reflects the reciprocal impacts of parenting on peer relations and of peer relations on subsequent parenting, as described in dynamic systems models (e.g., Granic & Patterson, 2006).

This dynamic developmental model describes, in part, how early risk is realized across time and also how each new developmental era affords new risk (and new opportunities for positive change). Importantly, it shows that risk of serious antisocial outcomes is probabilistic, and that it is premature to conclude that an early-starting aggressive 5-year-old is destined for a life-persistent path toward antisocial behavior and crime. Although the risk is substantial, our findings (and clinical experience) indicate that trajectories of risk can be deflected at multiple points in development through skill-building efforts and supportive interactions with parents, peers, school, and other important adults along the way. Accordingly, preventive intervention at key points in the life course can deflect high-risk children away from antisocial outcomes and future violence.

Although the Fast Track findings validate the developmental cascade model, it is also critical to recognize the enormous heterogeneity and individual differences evident in children's pathways to adolescent violence. This heterogeneity is best demonstrated by the findings described in Chapter 8 using person-oriented analyses. These analyses revealed that about one-third of the children in the high-risk control group who showed elevated aggression at school entry had no convictions in adolescence and early adulthood and another 10% showed the adolescent-limited profile of juvenile but no adult convictions (Goulter et al., 2018). Furthermore, among the youth who demonstrated persistent antisocial behavior through early adulthood, the strength of the factors that influenced their outcomes showed significant variation. The sample varied in markers of genetic risk and in the levels of adversity experienced in home and school settings. For some youth, risky behaviors in adolescence such as school failure and substance use escalated their pathways to criminal activity, whereas for others, these associated behaviors played a lesser role. We have been humbled at numerous times when our predictions regarding which children in Fast Track would have the worst outcomes were not realized, and children who we felt were at much less risk turned out to have very poor outcomes. We have all learned greater respect for how trauma or unexpected positive events throughout the developmental period can substantially change children's trajectories in unexpected ways.

## IMPLICATIONS FOR FUTURE PREVENTIVE INTERVENTIONS

Our tests of the developmental model and our intervention outcomes have several implications for future prevention efforts. First, they suggest that although each new developmental period may bring new risks that increase a child's risk for violent outcomes, it also provides new opportunities to change the child's developmental trajectory. For example, the quality of parenting that the child receives during early childhood, especially the supports that build social-emotional skills and address conduct problem behaviors may compensate for other aspects of an adverse environment. Similarly, effective SEL curricula and academic curricula at school may compensate for poor school readiness. Likewise, a difficult early school experience that places a child at risk for adolescent violence can be partially offset by parents who closely monitor and supervise their child and communicate with him or her during the course of adolescence. Each developmental phase affords a new opportunity for targeted intervention in specific domains. Our findings highlight specific targets for prevention that are particularly relevant at specific phases of development. During the early elementary years, these include parenting interventions, child-focused SEL programming, and cognitive developmental supports. During adolescence, these include family interventions, mentoring, and identity/career development supports. A second implication is that because new risks arise with each new developmental phase, preventive intervention cannot be deemed "over" until the child has passed through adolescence. Finally, validating our intervention model, it appears that the most effective preventive interventions will boost children's social-emotional competencies and address multiple aspects of a child's family and school life across multiple phases of development.

In addition to the Fast Track findings, new implications for intervention design have emerged from other areas of related investigation. Looking back over the past 29 years, substantial and important changes in our understanding of the causal processes and mechanisms of developmental change associated with trajectories of aggression have emerged. Here we discuss a number of these mechanisms and reflect on what we have learned from both our quantitative and clinical experiences during Fast Track, and how these lessons might be incorporated into future interventions targeting childhood aggression.

### Promoting Competencies and Strengths

From the outset, the Fast Track intervention focused primarily on promoting strengths and protective factors across development to address risks. For example, Fast Track focused on promoting skills for effective parenting and nurturing new competencies in classroom teaching. Most importantly, we focused on promoting child skills in areas of emotion regulation, self-control, friendship making, and social problem solving. We have shown that these social competencies in the early elementary years predict important outcomes in adulthood (Jones, Greenberg, & Crowley, 2015). We have also shown that improvements in children's prosocial behavior and self-regulation capabilities, especially their ability to regulate their emotions, use effective problem-solving skills, and form positive relationships with others, played a key role in reducing their risk for later antisocial outcomes (Sorensen et al., 2016).

Although we had a strong conceptualization and measurement model for the child skills targeted in the early elementary years, the skills we targeted in early adolescence were not as clearly or comprehensively conceptualized. With the advent of early adolescence, more advanced social-cognitive skills become important for self-control and decision making, as do a set of attitudes and motivational sets associated with identity formation and future goal attainment. In the years following Fast Track, recent and exciting developments in positive youth development and adolescent motivation suggest additional strategies that might have strengthened the prevention program impact in adolescence.

Fast Track incorporated mentoring, included workshops focused on components of Oyserman's model of "future selves" and related life skills, and provided career advising and support in small-group and individual meetings (Oyserman et al., 2002). However, more could have been done. For example, Damon (2008) and others have described experiences that contribute to the development of a sense of purpose in adolescence and strategies for promoting character, moral identity, and the capacity for useful engagement. In particular, reflective experiences with service learning may strengthen youth's positive connections to their communities and to positive role-model adults and foster a sense of personal pride and responsibility for improving life in their neighborhoods (Flanagan & Galley, 2014). A more comprehensive prevention program might have included these strategies.

Recent research on fostering growth mindsets in adolescents may also have enriched the Fast Track adolescent-phase intervention (Paunesku et al., 2015). When youth face new challenges or difficulties (such as transitions into new school settings or coping with poor grades), researchers have found that fostering normative thinking (e.g., many youth have similar experiences and feelings), growth beliefs (e.g., things can change for the better with problem solving and effort), and goal setting promote resilience and coping efforts, resulting in improved performance (Yeager et al., 2014). Including these strategies in the adolescent phase of the Fast Track intervention might have further nurtured positive goals and attitudes and sparked "healthy passions" during a period marked by strong negative peer influences and the rapid development of delinquent behavior.

## Neuropsychological Deficits and Implications for Intervention

Since the Fast Track program started in 1990, extensive research has identified neurocognitive processes that influence children's social-emotional development and behavioral adjustment (e.g., Ellis, Weiss, & Lochman, 2009) and that are linked with children's conduct problems (Matthys, Vanderschuren, Schutter, & Lochman, 2012). A key example involves children's reward sensitivity—their responses to reward and punishment. Most children feel pleasure, pride, and satisfaction when they are rewarded for particular behaviors, which then motivates them to perform the appropriate and socially desired behaviors that elicit rewards. Conversely, most children feel distressed, guilty, or embarrassed when they receive negative feedback and punishment, which helps them learn to inhibit the aggressive impulses and inappropriate behaviors that elicit those negative consequences. Emerging studies of children with conduct problems suggest that many have low sensitivity to reward and punishment cues, which impedes the social control of their aggression.

A parallel line of research has identified a subgroup of aggressive youth who show callous-unemotional (CU) traits—a lack of empathy for others' feelings and a lack of guilt for their own transgressions (for a review, see Frick, Ray, Thornton, & Kahn, 2014). These youth are at increased risk for poor outcomes in adolescence and adulthood (e.g., delinquency, juvenile and adult arrests, antisocial personality disorder), even after controlling for co-occuring conduct problems (McMahon, Witkiewitz, Kotler, & CPPRG, 2010). Thought to be genetic in basis and elicited when children face developmental adversity, youth with conduct problems and CU traits have low sensitivity to punishment cues and they appear particularly nonresponsive to harsh, critical parenting, although they respond to warm parenting (Pardini, Lochman & Powell, 2007; Pasalich et al., 2016).

Aggressive children who show low sensitivity to punishment or elevated CU traits may need tailored intervention strategies. For example, these children may require more extensive use of positive socialization supports with a reduced reliance on negative consequences or punishment. Accordingly, more time could be spent with parents and teachers on the use of relationship-building activities, clearly stated instructions and guidance, and praise and point systems with rewards. To strengthen the salience of these cues, particularly for children with comorbid inattention, it may help for parents and teachers to use touch and eye contact when providing instructions and delivering positive reinforcement (Dadds, Cauchi, Wimalaweera, Hawes, & Brennan, 2012). Likewise, the positive emotion associated with praise and reinforcement can be emphasized by expressing verbal and nonverbal enthusiasm during delivery. To increase children's attention to rewards, shorter behavioral monitoring intervals and more frequent and more salient rewards may help motivate children to strive toward their behavioral goals during intervention and in classroom and home settings. A recent study by Dadds and colleagues (2012) suggests that children with elevated CU traits may also benefit from extra supports and training in areas of emotion recognition and emotional understanding, as well as an emphasis on positive parenting (also see McMahon et al., 2018).

## The Role of Cognitive Control

Advances in developmental neuroscience since 1990 have identified the particularly important role that cognitive control processes play in reducing reactive aggression by supporting emotion regulation, attention control, and flexible problem solving. Research has identified a negative impact of early adversity on the development of children's executive functions, affecting children's attention skills, inhibitory control, working memory, and planning/decision-making skills (Blair & Raver, 2015). As a result, children and adolescents may have difficulty learning to regulate their reactions to frustration or provocation in order to optimize their behavior (that is, shift ideas, revise plans). Children with less well-developed executive functions often show poor impulse control and emotion regulation, both of which may fuel reactive aggression. Similarly, difficulties in planning ahead or anticipating negative outcomes may increase risk-taking behavior.

For children with poor executive-function skills, preventive intervention might be modified to provide additional training in areas of self-regulation and social problem-solving skills across the period of late childhood and early adolescence. Currently, few evidence-based interventions have demonstrated the capacity to improve executive-function skills and reduce associated emotional or behavioral regulation difficulties, but a number of approaches appear promising (see reviews by Bierman & Torres, 2016; Diamond & Lee, 2011). Components of cognitive control training might be particularly useful for these children and could be introduced in a group or individually. This training might include teaching children greater self-regulatory control, helping them to slow down in their cognitive process in order to better understand their social dilemmas, set positive goals to guide positive solutions to interpersonal problems, consider the potential consequences of different actions, and shift their plans based on feedback. This kind of approach has proven helpful for children with ADHD who often have deficits in executive-function skills (see Pfiffner et al., 2016).

Research shows that most intervention programs for aggressive children, including Fast Track, produce only modest effect sizes. Understanding the role of impaired neurocognitive functions in the social-learning processes of disruptive behavior problems may inform and improve interventions for these children. This focus may lead to a next wave of "mechanism" studies in prevention research. This focus might occur in at least two ways. First, the value of further training on self-regulation and executive-function skills could be evaluated. Second, personalized interventions could be evaluated, with components adjusted based upon the weaknesses and strengths of the child's neurocognitive characteristics associated with their social-learning difficulties.

## Mindfulness, Impulsivity, and Rumination

In addition to problems with self-control that are associated with impulsive behavior, many children with conduct problems also display comorbid depression or anxiety, especially as they move into the teen years and experience negative social outcomes (Odgers et al., 2007). During the past decade, promising findings have emerged in interventions that embed mindfulness practices for adults (and sometimes children), designed to help individuals become more aware of their thoughts, feelings, and behaviors, and to slow down cognitive processes and associated difficulties such as ruminative thoughts.

Mindfulness is the practice of bringing nonjudgmental awareness to the present moment, and is derived from Buddhist and other contemplative practices (Kabat-Zinn, 1990). A growing body of evidence with adults demonstrates that mindfulness promotes psychological well-being by teaching skills that improve attentional capacity and self-regulation of emotions, cognition, and behavior (Hölzel et al., 2011). Studies with adults show positive effects of mindfulness on reductions in depression, anxiety, pain, and insomnia and increases in enhanced immune functioning (Goyal et al., 2014). Mindfulness practices have been associated with enhanced emotional self-regulation and attentional control in adults (Creswell, Way, Eisenberger, & Lieberman, 2007; Tang et al., 2007).

Several theorists have suggested that impulsivity and emotion dysregulation, particularly reactive aggression, may benefit from training in mindfulness practices in ways that are not well-treated by other cognitive behavioral intervention strategies alone. Compared to other forms of aggression, reactive aggression has distinct physiological correlates, including intense autonomic arousal and activation of the HPA axis, that suggest it is motivated, in part, by stress reactivity (Lopez-Duran, Olson, Hajal, Felt, & Vazquez, 2009). Children who exhibit high rates of reactive aggression show heightened reactivity to interpersonal rejection (Hubbard et al., 2002) and difficulty reducing arousal following provocation (Williams, Lochman, Phillips, & Barry, 2003). Learning to reduce this reactivity may be important for later aggression control. Consistent with this hypothesis, Carre and colleagues (2014) tested a subsample of predominantly black males who participated in Fast Track and found that, at age 26, those who were in the intervention group demonstrated reduced testosterone reactivity to social provocations that, in turn, mediated the intervention effect on reduced aggression.

There is a limited research base for mindfulness practices but a recent meta-analysis of programs for youth suggest some promising effects on improved social competence, anger control, and reduced inattention, anxiety, and rumination (Carsley, Khoury & Heath, 2018; Mind and Life Education Research Network, 2012). To date, meta-analyses do not support the effectiveness of mindfulness programs in reducing aggressive behavior when implemented in the classroom (Maynard, Solis, Miller, & Brendel, 2017), but suggest that mindfulness components may strengthen individual treatments for aggressive children with developmental disabilities (Klingbeil et al., 2017). Several small studies show that children with aggressive and disruptive behavior problems respond favorably to mindfulness strategies and these may be particularly useful in early adolescence as children become more aware of their thoughts and how they affect their behavior (Bögels, Hoogstad, van Dun, de Schutter, & Resifo, 2008; Singh et al., 2007). For children who are quite active and impulsive, interventions that combine physical yoga with more traditional mindfulness practices (silent meditations verbally led by a teacher at the end of yoga in the corpse/savasana position) may be optimal (see Frank & Bose, 2014; Mendelson et al., 2013). However, high-quality randomized-controlled trials with follow-up assessments are needed to determine the utility of mindfulness practices for highly aggressive children (Greenberg & Harris, 2012).

Fostering mindfulness in parents (mindful parenting) may increase positive parenting (Dumas, 2005) by improving parents' own self-regulation, lowering their emotional reactivity and increasing their warmth and compassion for their children (Duncan, Coatsworth, & Greenberg, 2009). Mindfulness strategies for parents include a specific focus on increasing parents' awareness of parenting-related thoughts, feelings, and behaviors. In addition, mindfulness practices encourage parents to be more "present" and attentive with their children, as well as to be more intentional and compassionate (Bögels & Restifo, 2014). This may help parents regulate their own responses in parent–child inter-changes and focus on building warm, positive connections with their child. In one study, mindfulness strategies were infused into a univer-sal family-based preventive intervention designed to reduce adolescent substance use, the Strengthening Families Program (Coatsworth et al., 2015). Adding the mindfulness component increased impact on posi-tive parenting practices relative to the standard Strengthening Families Program, leading to greater improvements in parent anger-management skills, parent–child relationship quality, and consistent discipline. Simi-larly, a theoretically informed, developmentally sensitive integration of mindfulness strategies into existing evidence-based cognitive behavioral interventions for children with aggressive behavior has led to improved emotional and behavioral regulation (Miller et al., 2018) and might have been incorporated into Fast Track had we begun this work more recently. It will be important for future research to both understand the impact of mindful parenting and mindful programs for highly aggressive children at high risk for CD, as well as to explore whether mindfulness strategies can be infused into existing comprehensive preventive inter-vention for these children.

## Genetics and Epigenetics

We began Fast Track before the "genetics revolution." Sequencing the human genome has fostered increased understanding of the ongoing transactional processes that link genetic and environmental influences on development and functioning. Translational epigenetics research has enriched models describing changes in gene activation associated with exposure to and reaction to stress (Cole, 2013; Fredrickson et al., 2015; Meany, 2001). Although genes were once considered static and nonmalleable, recent research suggests that environmental factors often regulate gene expression, essentially turning them on and off. This work has shown that one way in which adverse environments may confer risk for negative outcomes is through sustained epigenetic modifications—in other words, changing the ways in which genes are expressed. If this is the case, then one question is whether *positive* environmental influ-ences, such as those produced by intervention programs, can also pro-duce epigenetic effects and reverse the negative effects of adverse envi-ronments (e.g., Perroud et al., 2013; Yehuda et al., 2013). For example, Roberts and colleagues (2014) found that increases in methylation in the promoter region of the serotonin transporter was associated with better response to cognitive behavioral therapy in children with anxiety disorders.

The availability of genetic information for youth in the Fast Track sample has permitted a set of exploratory studies designed to better understand the environmental conditions under which genetic risk factors related to poor outcomes are expressed and possibly affected by intervention. For example, as described in Chapter 8, the glucocorticoid receptor plays a critical role in the human stress response as it influences short- and long-term adaptations of the HPA axis to environmental challenge and stress (Meany, 2001). Variation in the glucocorticoid receptor gene *NR3C1* moderated Fast Track intervention impact for white children (Albert, Belsky, Crowley, Latendresse, et al., 2015), with 18% of Fast Track children as compared to 75% of control children showing externalizing psychopathology at age 25 follow-up among those carrying the A allele. In another study, Zheng and colleagues (2018) found that, among the black youth carrying the minor allele of the *NR3C1* single-nucleotide polymorphism (*rs12655166*), intervention was more effective at reducing linear growth in alcohol abuse during adolescence compared to those without the minor allele.

While these gene × intervention moderation effects need to be replicated, they support theoretical models that indicate that children who show the most genetic vulnerability to the negative effects of adversity may also be most likely to show positive outcomes when they receive enriched environments (Ellis, Boyce, Belsky, Bakermans-Kranenburg, & van IJzendoorn, 2011). From this perspective, society's glaring failure to provide basic social and emotional supports to disadvantaged children not only increases the probability that some will develop chronic conduct problems, but also neglects a critical opportunity to promote positive, healthy development.

Finally, these gene × intervention moderation findings have important implications for the conceptualization of preventive interventions. First, they illustrate the importance of developmental timing. Fast Track already began to "interrupt" the effects of genetic risk on externalizing behaviors by third grade and thus allowed for fewer dysfunctional effects associated with the negative cascade of misbehavior, rejection, and alienation (Albert, Belsky, Crowley, Bates, et al., 2015). However, the fact that we found further gene × intervention interaction effects in adolescence suggests that it might be *necessary but not sufficient* to address disruptive behavior in childhood. Children with heightened biological sensitivity to social stressors are likely to be particularly vulnerable to social-emotional disruption at major developmental transitions such as puberty and entry into secondary school. It would be unwise to assume that successful prevention of conduct problems in elementary school will completely buffer children from the challenges and risks of adolescence (Moffitt, 1993).

These studies represent an early step in understanding the complicated pathways through which genetic phenotypes may affect response to a psychosocial intervention and may thereby inform intervention tailoring. Testing for gene × intervention effects in prevention trials both provides a means for evaluating these pathways of influence and informs the design and refinement of intervention models (Brody et al., 2013). Results from this type of gene × intervention research may lead to small, efficient trials (microtrials) that target individuals with specific genotypes or test more narrowly defined interventions and outcomes, or both (Collins et al., 2011). A second stage of full-scale studies might then test multiple intervention variables and outcome measures simultaneously to examine synergies and interferences among the intervention components. For a complex behavior such as a response to a psychosocial intervention, we anticipate that the action of many loci would be involved—leading to genetic risk being distributed along a broad continuum.

## ISSUES ABOUT INTERVENTION STRUCTURE AND FORMAT

### Peer Effects in Group Interventions

Despite the positive effects of Fast Track and other group-based cognitive behavioral interventions, it is critical to respond to concerns and findings that interventions that aggregate high-risk children into groups might be potentially iatrogenic (Dishion, McCord, & Poulin, 1999; Dishion, Dodge, & Lansford, 2006). Developmental research has indicated that children with problem behavior are likely to affiliate with each other and that involvement with deviant peers leads to increased risk for adolescent problem behaviors (Arnold & Hughes, 1999). As a result of deviant-peer effects, group interventions have the potential to escalate or maintain, rather than reduce, youth behavior problems. Research about deviant-peer influences has been sufficiently worrisome to suggest caution in aggregating high-risk youth in clinical, educational, or correctional settings (Dodge et al., 2006; Poulin, Dishion, & Burraston, 2001). However, meta-analytic research has not found evidence that group interventions for disruptive youth lead to iatrogenic deviancy training effects (e.g., Lipsey, 2006; Weiss et al., 2005), nor were any iatrogenic effects evident in the Fast Track Friendship Groups (Lavallee et al., 2005). Although many agree that the potential for deviancy training in group interventions for disruptive youth *may* occur, there has been a lack of well-controlled studies to clarify the conditions under which iatrogenic effects are most likely to emerge.

The first intervention study to draw attention to the potential harm of the peer context of an intervention was in the St. Louis Experiment (Feldman et al., 1983). Similarly, the Cambridge–Somerville Youth

Study reported iatrogenic effects on adult adjustment as a function of randomization to the multicomponent intervention condition (McCord, 1992). Youth who were sent to summer camps with other aggressive youth showed a 10-fold increased likelihood of negative life outcomes (criminal behavior, alcoholism, mental health problems) in comparison to control youth.

In a more recent study, the Adolescent Transitions Program, which involved cognitive-behavioral youth groups focusing on self-regulation, demonstrated improvements in observed family interaction; however, the intervention also led to increases in youth reports of smoking and teacher reports of problem behavior at school at 1-year and 3-year follow-ups (Dishion & Andrews, 1995; Poulin et al., 2001). Analyses of the iatrogenic group conditions revealed that subtle dynamics of deviancy training during unstructured transitions in the groups predicted growth in self-reported smoking and teacher ratings of delinquency (Dishion, Poulin, & Burraston., 2001). Group effects were minimal, and negative outcomes in the intervention seemed largely attributable to individuals dispersed across groups. This and other research suggest that appropriate placement of different subtypes of youth in intervention contexts may be the best strategy for optimizing intervention effectiveness and minimizing harm.

Although there are concerns about deviant-peer effects in interventions for children with conduct problems, there are also important potential benefits to using a group delivery format, thus making decisions about intervention delivery complex. First, working with children in groups is more cost-effective than individually delivered intervention (Mager, Milich, Harris, & Howard, 2005; Manassis et al., 2002). This is an important consideration at all levels of mental health service delivery, as cost-effectiveness may enhance the broader use of a program. Second, group reward systems and peer reinforcement can play an important role in assisting children to attain intervention-related goals and thus to generalize behavioral improvements resulting from the intervention to children's real-world school and home settings (Poulin et al., 2001). Third, groups can permit children to develop prosocial leadership skills (Flannery-Schroeder & Kendall, 2000). Fourth, the group format may be less threatening to children with conduct problems than an individual program that singles them out, especially in the school setting (Schechtman & Ben-David, 1999). Fifth, the group format permits children to practice learned skills in social interaction (Poulin et al., 2001) and the small-group format has generally been considered better than the individual format for skills training (Landau, Milich, & Diener, 1998). Inclusion of peers in small-group interventions facilitates opportunities for practice of social and emotional skills, allows children to receive peer feedback about social and emotional skill performance, and fosters children's abilities to generalize use of skills with peers (Bierman, 1986; Lavallee et al., 2005). Intervention techniques such as role playing, peer modeling, and peer reinforcement of adaptive behavior can only be accomplished in small-group formats (Mager et al., 2005).

Despite the importance of this issue, there have been few studies that have explored group versus individual formats with the same intervention for children. A recently conducted study carefully compared group versus individual formats for the Coping Power Program on subsequent adjustment outcomes in early adolescent youth (Lochman et al., 2015). Growth curve analyses indicated that aggressive children with poor inhibitory control showed significantly greater reductions over time on teacher-rated measures of adjustment (externalizing and internalizing problems, deviant-peer involvement) when treated individually rather than in a group context. These more impulsive aggressive children may have been more susceptible to negative peer influence in the group setting. Aggressive children who were more socially oriented, as indexed by the G allele of an oxytocin receptor gene single-nucleotide polymorphism (Glenn et al., 2018), and who had greater difficulty regulating their emotional recovery following frustration, as indexed by respiratory sinus arrhythmia activity in the parasympathetic nervous system (Glenn et al., 2019), showed greater teacher-rated improvement when seen in the individual-intervention format than in the group-intervention format. These findings underscore the need for future research exploring the types of children who may respond better to individual versus group interventions to reduce aggression.

In addition, the characteristics of effective group programs require further study. That is, data are needed to clarify how group leaders can best manage group sessions to reduce deviancy training during sessions. Studies of Coping Power groups, which included observations of 938 group sessions, showed that group leaders who used effective behavior management strategies and timely delivery of program elements, in conjunction with a warm, nonirritable clinical style produced the best child outcomes (Lochman et al., 2017). Thus, it will be crucially important to engage in rigorous research to better understand the potential effects of group versus individual interventions when coupled with optimal training for group leaders. Perhaps strong program organization and training may reduce risk for deviant-peer effects in group settings, thereby allowing for more cost-effective group interventions.

## Linking and Integrating Universal and Targeted Interventions

The primary aim of the Fast Track project was to develop, implement, and evaluate a comprehensive intervention to prevent severe and chronic conduct problems in a sample of children selected at high risk when they first entered school. In doing so, we hoped to demonstrate the value of a comprehensive prevention model that combined universal and indicated intervention into an integrated set of activities. This is a rare event, as these two different approaches to universal (primary) and indicated and targeted (secondary) prevention emerged from different conceptual traditions and are rarely combined (Greenberg & Riggs, 2015; Weissberg & Greenberg, 1998).

There are two central reasons why the integrated delivery of universal and indicated interventions should provide an additive effect. First, it is unlikely that effects of the indicated interventions with high-risk children and families will generalize to the school and classroom setting without providing support for these new skills in the school (Kazdin, 1993). By providing similar skills, cues, and a common language in both the indicated and universal interventions, teachers and other school staff are prepared to promote the generalization of skills to the classroom, playground, and peer interactions. Second, a universal intervention intended to promote the development of social competence in all children should lead to an improved classroom atmosphere that supports improved interpersonal relations for all students (Battistich, Solomon, Watson, Solomon, & Schaps, 1989). Indeed, our findings on the classroom effects of the universal curriculum showed that it had broad effects on teacher reports of behavior and sociometric status through grade 3 (CPPRG, 1999b, 2010c). Reciprocally, more intensive intervention with the highest-risk children in these same classrooms may serve to reduce their highly disruptive impact on the classrooms, and thus make it easier for the remaining children to respond to the universal intervention.

At the time, Fast Track was unique in combining interventions at the universal and targeted level. Since then, conceptual models in prevention science, special education, and school psychology all favor the integration of universal, selective, and indicated levels of intervention intensity (Sanders, 2012; Stephan, Sugai, Lever, & Connors, 2015). Additional examples of model programs demonstrate the feasibility and potential power of tiered prevention supports and integrating school-based and parent-focused interventions (Bierman, Heinrichs, Welsh, Nix, & Gest, 2017; Pfiffner et al., 2016). Challenges continue, however, in the implementation of multitiered programs (Kratochwill, Volpiansky, Clements, & Ball, 2007), documenting the need for additional research in this area.

## Enhancing Intervention Engagement

Despite positive outcome results for Fast Track, we experienced substantial challenges in program implementation (McGowan, Nix, Murphy, Bierman, & CPPRG, 2010). Substantial difficulties in program implementation have also been noted in other preadolescent and adolescent interventions (Boxmeyer, Lochman, Powell, Windle, & Wells, 2008; Durlak & DuPre, 2008). A key implementation concern involves the difficulty in successfully engaging some parents and youth in preventive intervention, and once engaged, maintaining their active involvement and engagement (Lochman, Powell, Jackson, & Czopp, 2006).

Since the initiation of Fast Track, technology-based communication systems have advanced considerably, making possible the use of a wide variety of multimedia materials and technology-based strategies to enhance participant engagement (and outcomes) in programs (for reviews, see Anton & Jones, 2017; MacDonell & Prinz, 2017). Technology-based interventions have been widely advocated in the fields of health education and prevention (Lightfoot, Rotheram-Borus, Comulada, Reddy, & Duan, 2010), as Internet delivery potentially permits interventions to be more accessible (Taylor et al., 2008), more efficient and less burdensome (Bishop, Bryant, Giles, Hansen, & Dusenbury, 2006), and ultimately more cost efficient. Technology-based interventions include both stand-alone and technology-enhanced interventions. The former refers to those technology-based interventions that do not involve any clinician contact (e.g., self-guided mobile apps, Internet-based treatments), whereas the latter involve some level of therapist involvement (e.g., video teleconferencing, telephone support; Anton & Jones, 2017). There is emerging evidence that family-based interventions delivered via the Internet, either as stand-alone programs (e.g., Sanders, Baker, & Turner, 2012), via videoconferencing to remotely deliver parent management training (Comer et al., 2017), or as adjuncts to clinic-delivered (e.g., Jones, Forehand, Cuellar, Parent, & Honeycutt, 2014) and school-delivered (Lochman, Boxmeyer et al., 2017) interventions are effective with a variety of families of children with conduct problems (see reviews by Breitenstein, Gross, & Christophersen, 2014; McGoron & Ondersma, 2015; MacDonell & Prinz, 2017). As one recent example, an Internet version of Parent–Child Interaction Therapy (I-PCIT) provided stronger effects on some outcomes than therapist-delivered PCIT (Comer et al., 2017; Comer, 2015).

Researchers are now drawing attention to various challenges and issues involved in the uptake and implementation of technology-based interventions (e.g., Anton & Jones, 2017; Chou, Bry, & Comer, 2017), and Anton and Jones have provided a conceptual framework for facilitating uptake and implementation of technology-enhanced treatments by individual therapists as well as provider organizations. These novel approaches to the delivery of family-based interventions for CD hold promise for increasing the reach of such interventions to families (e.g., those in rural or underresourced communities) who may not typically receive them.

Existing evidence suggests face-to-face contact is important to keep parents engaged in parenting interventions and blended models (face-to-face combined with technology-assisted) may be more effective at engaging parents than technology-assisted alone (Hall & Bierman, 2015). Although Internet delivery of interventions may be sufficient in providing simple information that can help to alleviate mild or concrete problems, the personal assistance of a clinician in a hybrid intervention delivery model may be important in modifying more significant, stable behavioral habits such as aggression. For example, Taylor and colleagues (2008) used a hybrid model of the Incredible Years program that combined computer and web-based delivery of information and video-modeling vignettes along with direct professional intervention through home visits and phone calls. When employed with Head Start families, this hybrid model led to a high level of parental satisfaction with the program and to an increased completion rate, with 76% completing the entire program and 82% completing at least half. In another example, Jones and colleagues (2014) presented preliminary evidence that a technology-enhanced version of Helping the Noncompliant Child (HNC; McMahon & Forehand, 2003) utilizing a smartphone app that included an HNC skills video series, brief daily surveys, text-message reminders, video recording of home practice, and midweek video calls enhanced engagement and outcome, compared to HNC alone, for a sample of economically disadvantaged families.

Hybrid Internet intervention programs can potentially be delivered with fewer face-to-face sessions than with traditional versions of the same program, and thus may be briefer and promote greater implementation feasibility. To avoid barriers, preventive interventionists in schools can use an implementation and sustainability framework that addresses the fit between the demands of an intervention and the school context (Forman, Olin, Hoagwood, Crowe, & Saka, 2009). Lengthy interventions can be perceived to be a problem in the school context because they can be perceived to interfere with school policies and demands, and because the results may not be immediately observed at the end of the intervention. With targeted preadolescent aggressive children, a recent feasibility study has found that an Internet hybrid version of the Coping Power Program could be delivered with 60% fewer face-to-face sessions (Lochman, Boxmeyer, et al., 2017). It was enthusiastically received by children, and produced reductions in teacher-rated conduct problems, in comparison to an untreated control group.

Thus, there are several implications for the use of technology in future prevention research for programs like Fast Track. Some training of SEL concepts can be conducted through websites accessed by children and by parents, thus permitting face-to-face sessions to be more focused on the application of those skills. Children's and parents' use of interesting material on the websites can deepen their level of engagement with the intervention and increase their likelihood of attending future face-to-face sessions. Personal intervention-related online chats between staff and the participants can especially deepen children's and parents' levels of clinical engagement with the intervention staff. Future programs can also provide media-based text reminders and parenting messages to remind children and parents about new skills and tasks and to reinforce their use of these skills. The content of the material delivered via technology would necessarily need to change, and become more sophisticated, as children developed.

## ISSUES IN HETEROGENEITY, TAILORING, AND EFFICIENCY

### Tailoring Intervention to Promote Family Engagement

Family involvement in educational and mental health services is critical for children with conduct problems (for reviews, see Chacko et al., 2016; Piotrowska et al., 2017). Benefits of family involvement include higher academic achievement, increased parent support of teachers and schools, and increased likelihood of enrolling in postsecondary education programs (e.g., Epstein, 1991; Henderson & Mapp, 2002).

As noted in prior chapters, we used a number of procedures to promote parental engagement in Fast Track. These procedures ranged from providing transportation to parent meetings, holding parent meetings in community settings (often in the neighborhood school) near where people lived, serving snacks, providing supervised child monitoring during parent meetings to assist parents who had siblings who were younger (or even older) than the Fast Track target children, and paying parents for their time participating in group sessions. We also attempted to recruit diverse FCs from the communities we worked in who were sensitive to parents' community contexts and cultural histories and who could form strong working relationships with parents (e.g. Orrell-Valente et al., 1999). With these intensive engagement procedures, we achieved relatively high levels of parental attendance, especially in the early years of elementary school. However, a subset of parents never, or only rarely, participated in the parent intervention. For some of these parents, low group attendance reflected a preference for individual home visits, which were conducted whenever possible when parents missed a group session (Nix et al., 2009). However, in other cases, low group attendance reflected a general disengagement with Fast Track. For this reason, building parent engagement strategies into existing practices and programs can be seen as an essential goal for the delivery of high-quality services in schools.

A platform such as the Family Check Up (FCU; Dishion & Storm-shak, 2007) is one example of a parental engagement tool that can be integrated into existing interventions. FCU uses an initial assessment and feedback session to provide parents with information about child and family strengths and risk factors. The FCU feedback session is intended to help motivate families to take advantage of intervention opportunities and to become more involved in their children's lives. The clinician prepares a single-page feedback form, based on assessments from family and school sources, to highlight areas of strength as well as areas of concern during the meeting. During the meeting, the clinician uses a motivational interviewing approach and strategies to facilitate the discussion and to elicit motivational talk from the parent. Parents can perceive that the clinician recognizes their personal and social strengths and their desire for a positive outcome for their children, while collab-oratively exploring problem areas that exist in the family and child that could become the focus of intervention. An FCU feedback session ends with the development of an action plan about next steps based on the needs highlighted in the feedback discussion. The emphasis on providing parents with intervention options is a key part of the procedure. The par-ent and clinician can then decide on a jointly tailored set of intervention goals directly targeting the identified child and family problem areas. Previous research indicates that the FCU increases parent engagement and leads to reliable reductions in problem behavior in children and ado-lescents (Boyd-Ball & Dishion, 2006; Connell, Dishion, Yasui, & Kava-nagh, 2007). Further, the families most in need of family intervention services (e.g., single parents, those from high-conflict homes, those with deviant-peer involvement) engage more consistently in the FCU.

Conceptually, the FCU could be integrated with an evidence-based program, like Fast Track, for children with conduct problems. In that case, the feedback session could lead to a discussion about which ses-sions and components the parent would like to complete and in what order (Herman et al., 2012). The core components of the evidence-based program could be identified and separated into different modules (e.g., stress management; instructions, rules, and expectations; limit setting) that parents could select to work on in any sequence. For example, in creating an action plan for next steps, a parent may elect to focus on a stress-management module first before beginning on a parenting tool kit, based on feedback the parent receives about assessments of their stress and depression levels. Future research could test whether a tra-ditional intervention such as Fast Track might be infused with moti-vational interviewing and FCU principles, which could then lead to effective, briefer, and tailored interventions for at-risk children and their parents.

On a related front, the recent presentation of a comprehensive process model of parental engagement in treatment (CAPE; Piotrowska et al., 2017) provides an excellent heuristic framework for future research in this area. The elements include Connect and Attend (i.e., enrollment and attendance), Participate (which includes in-session discussion and homework completion), and Enact (implementation of the newly learned parenting strategies).

## Understanding the Intervention Response

The purpose of individualizing or tailoring multicomponent interventions is twofold: (1) to increase participant engagement by aligning intervention focus with participant goals and preferences, and (2) to focus the intervention specifically on areas of individual child and family need. Conceptually, tailored interventions have the capacity to provide more efficient intervention than standard interventions (Collins, Murphy, & Bierman, 2004). At the same time, tailored interventions assume a certain level of specificity in the underlying prevention science, based on the expectation that particular components or modules address domain-specific needs. The Fast Track findings suggest some domain-specificity that supports this conceptualization. For example, improvements in the academic domain did not mediate improvements in aggressive behavior; developmental trajectories involving academic skills and social-emotional behavior appeared independent (CPPRG, 2004a). This suggests that interventions in these domains might also be independent and that academic tutoring could be provided only to children with academic needs without reducing the overall impact of the prevention program. We believe that this new understanding would alter the design of intervention for these children. At the same time, it is less clear whether the prevention program could be effective at reducing child and adolescent antisocial activity without including parent-focused components, even if a child's conduct problems occur primarily at school. This is because, based on the developmental model, parents play a key role in monitoring and supervising behaviors that create the opportunities for antisocial behavior.

# Chapter 10

# How Can Communities Address the Problem of Future Violence by Focusing on High-Risk Young Children?

This chapter is intended for those readers who are interested in developing prevention programs that will reduce the problem of violence in children who are most at risk. This goal requires a shift in focus from much of the rest of this volume, which focused on a standardized preventive intervention involving a rigorous, randomized controlled trial evaluation. Some decisions that we made in designing the Fast Track prevention program were constrained by the need to implement a standard set of procedures across four very different communities and to follow specific groups of children from kindergarten through high school and into adulthood. As reflected in this book, our approach provided rich information about the impact of the prevention program and the capacity to examine effects of the same program implemented in different contexts. On the other hand, communities interested in improving outcomes of children and families at high risk for future antisocial activity and violence need to focus on providing services that maximize effectiveness (and cost-effectiveness) within *their particular communities*. Hence, certain decisions made for Fast Track may require reconsideration in some community contexts.

The title of this chapter deliberately refers to *communities* as the active agent in making the decision to make a collaborative effort in reducing violence in their midst. *Community* can be defined in various ways and here we consider it to be the geographic area that bounds a school catchment area or a series of schools that are geographically or structurally connected. Communities include school systems—superintendents, school boards, principals, and teachers—but also other agencies that may become involved in implementation. In looking back, we see that a sustained effort requires the ongoing commitment of the community. Fast Track project funding came as a large single grant from the federal government. It is difficult to envision that a similar financial decision could be made in current times. Even without this kind of federal support, we think it is possible for community leaders to take collective action to decide to combine and coordinate their resources in ways that can reduce youth violence in their community. We advocate collective action because the problems that high-risk children with conduct problems experience over time take a considerable financial toll on many local agencies (e.g., education, police, courts, physical and behavioral health care) that are primarily organized to alleviate the many facets of this problem as it is occurring, rather than to prevent the future frequency of its occurrence.

In this chapter, we reflect on the challenges associated with the design of cost-effective prevention programs for high-risk children and youth with conduct problems. Given that government agencies and other foundations are increasingly interested in funding evidence-based programs, we recommend the use of the core Fast Track prevention components in future programming. This recommendation does not mean that we minimize other programs that have been shown to be effective in dealing with factors in the development of conduct problems in childhood and adolescence. However, we think that our findings reflect the importance of an early-initiated and sustained implementation of school and family components that provide high-risk children with the social and emotional regulation skills that help them to be successful and effectively manage strong feelings and control their behavior. Likewise, we believe that parents must be supported to adopt effective and nurturing strategies to raise their children with the skills to deal with adverse environments. However, we also reflect on our experiences and recommend several "choice points" at which some modification of the Fast Track procedures is likely to improve the feasibility and cost-effectiveness of sustainable Fast Track prevention services at the community level. Before addressing the challenges and alternatives to be considered in adapting the Fast Track program, we reflect on what we have learned about prevention from the findings presented in this volume.

First, if one works with small numbers of children in a targeted manner, it is difficult to have significant impact on adolescent and young adult violence and crime unless the target population has a relatively high base rate of this disorder. Thus, for example, we did not have much impact altering young adult violence and crime in females, even though those selected for the intervention had risk scores entering first grade that were comparable to males. This is because female rates of violence and serious crime were quite low in later life. Therefore, in identifying the size of the high-risk sample, we recommend using a base rate that is similar to the rate of violence in the community population. That is, if the rate of young adult violent crime in the population is 10%, then the program should target the 10% of the population at highest risk. These two points suggest that a community planning a comprehensive prevention effort must have a relatively good estimate of their community's base rate for the behavior to be prevented and target that part of their population that exhibits the highest levels of risk for that behavior.

Second, the goal of intervention should be to prevent serious violent crime in young adulthood, recognizing that this goal is different from preventing minor delinquent acts in early adolescence. Adolescents living in and attending school in relatively high-risk neighborhoods are likely to engage in minor delinquent acts that may appear to be normative for the community group but can result in arrests. Boys of color living in disadvantaged neighborhoods are more likely to get arrested for minor delinquency than their more advantaged peers (Sampson, 2017). True high-risk outcomes, as measured by severity and frequency of offending, appear in later adolescence and young adulthood, and we have documented that these outcomes have been substantially reduced by the Fast Track intervention. This does not mean that communities should not attempt to reduce early adolescent offending. It just means that some of this behavior may be normative at this age in some communities and that the community goal should be to reduce repeated offending and escalation in the severity of offending.

Although communities may attempt to reduce violence in diverse ways, including policies or practices that address threats of violence such as gun control, police or neighborhood watch systems, or adolescent treatment programs targeting youth in trouble with the law, this chapter focuses specifically on the early prevention approach of the Fast Track program. That is, it focuses on how communities might implement a developmentally informed early prevention program based upon the Fast Track model to address the child skills, parenting/family factors, school context features, and peer influences associated with the escalation of early childhood conduct problems into persistent and severe antisocial activities and violence. Fast Track included both universal prevention components (i.e., the PATHS curriculum to enhance early SEL and a positive school climate) and targeted prevention components (i.e., the intensive academic, social-emotional, and family support services provided to children screened for high risk based on early conduct problems). This chapter focuses primarily on the design and delivery of these targeted prevention components. Critical issues discussed in the following sections include (1) the design of screening systems to identify children who need early prevention services; (2) the selection of staffing and delivery systems to provide the Fast Track prevention components of child social skill training groups, peer pairing, academic tutoring, mentoring, Parent Group training, and home visiting; and (3) tailoring the program to address community needs. Across these issues, we focus in particular on modifications that might improve the community integration and sustainability of the Fast Track prevention program components as well as its cost-effectiveness.

## SCREENING PROCEDURES

A critical challenge of any targeted prevention program is to determine how and when to identify the children who are at highest risk for antisocial outcomes, in order to focus prevention efforts where they are most needed. In Fast Track, we chose kindergarten as the optimal time to identify high-risk children for targeted prevention services. As was discussed in Chapter 7, there is good evidence that children can be identified as significantly at risk for chronic juvenile offending at this age, although the true positive rate is still only 50%. Reflecting on our experiences, the timing and nature of our screening procedures had both positive and nonoptimal features.

### Is Kindergarten the Right Time to Screen?

Screening to identify children and families for targeted Fast Track prevention services during kindergarten was based on both developmental science and practical considerations. From a developmental standpoint, problem behaviors such as impulsivity, noncompliance, and hitting are relatively common during early childhood and not necessarily indicative of chronic behavioral difficulties. Young children are developing the self-regulatory skills that allow them to follow rules and control their impulses. Hence, some of the children who appear hyperactive, disruptive, and aggressive in early childhood settle down as they mature and experience supportive socialization at home and in school. In general, the younger the age of the screening, the greater the likelihood that "false positives" will be identified—that is, children who appear at risk for conduct problems, but who will settle down and gain control over their behavior over time, without any additional intervention. On the other hand, the later the age of the screening, the more intractable the problems may be, and the greater the difficulty in mounting a successful prevention program. Hence, deciding on the optimal timing for screening and the initiation of the prevention programming requires careful consideration.

In the case of Fast Track, we were also focused on practical considerations with regard to population-based screening. That is, we were interested in doing a population-wide screening, to the extent possible, in order to serve as many of the high-risk children in the local communities as possible. Although signs of elevated conduct problems are often evident before kindergarten entry, screening in kindergarten offered us the best chance of screening the majority of children in a given community (i.e., all that were attending public school). Such comprehensive screening is more difficult prior to kindergarten because children are in a wide variety of early child-care settings or still at home.

Based on developmental science, we concluded that rates of conduct problems are stable enough by age 6 to make this age a reasonably good time at which to identify children who are on problematic developmental trajectories and to initiate prevention activities early in school when negative developmental cascades could be prevented. Children who show high rates of conduct problems in kindergarten often have additional adjustment problems that cause them trouble in the school setting, including social skill deficits, attention problems, and low levels of academic readiness. We reasoned that early identification in kindergarten would allow for a timely initiation of prevention activities to build competencies and thereby reduce risks of school maladjustment.

At the same time, we found that the stability of conduct problems when screened in kindergarten is not ideal for an intensive and sustained prevention program such as Fast Track because of the number of children who screen in as false positives and reduce their aggression over time without intervention. We subsequently found that we could significantly increase the rate of successful identification by testing children again toward the end of first grade (Hill et al., 2004). In reflecting on our solution, we believe that the end of the kindergarten year is a good time to conduct screening to identify children at risk who could benefit from prevention activities that begin at the start of first grade. However, we would *not* recommend conducting this screening at the start of the kindergarten year, when children are just entering the formal school context and getting adjusted to it. During the initial months of kindergarten, some children show a "honeymoon" period, in which they show few behavior problems when they are first settling into school. For these children, behavior problems may not emerge until a few months into the year when they have become more comfortable in the school setting. At the other end of the spectrum, some children show a "slow to warm up" pattern in which they appear more maladjusted during the initial months of school because they are getting acclimated to the school context and demands. These children may settle down a few months into the year. However, by midway through the kindergarten year, behavioral adjustment becomes more stable, and teachers are able to more accurately assess the degree to which children have ongoing difficulties with conduct problems. For these reasons, the Fast Track screen was conducted in the second half of the kindergarten year.

Even if one waits until later in the kindergarten year to conduct the screening, it will still be the case that some behavior problems will show developmental instability. In hindsight, we believe that it would have been useful to repeat the screen toward the middle of first grade, in order to allow children who had established behavioral control by first grade to "graduate" out of the prevention program early. Our findings suggest that there was reduced value-added in keeping children with lower screen scores in the long-term prevention program, because these children were substantially less likely to become involved in violent crime over time, and hence did not need the intensive and costly prevention programming from which higher-risk children benefitted.

### Are Both Teacher and Parent Ratings Needed for This Screen?

A second feature of our screen score that made it more challenging to implement was the use of a two-gate screen that included parent ratings as well as teacher ratings. Our subsequent analyses suggested that the inclusion of parent ratings increased the precision of the kindergarten teacher screen. However, the added value was rather small, and when first-grade teacher ratings were used, there was no added advantage of collecting ratings from parents. From an administrative standpoint, it is clearly easier to conduct a screen that involves only teacher ratings. Our findings suggest that teachers are fairly good at identifying the highest-risk children, particularly if both kindergarten and first-grade teachers provide ratings.

For most schools and communities, relying on teachers to identify children who qualify for prevention makes a population-based screening much more feasible than trying to include parents in the screening process. Clearly, parental input and involvement is critical for effective prevention—but this input may not be needed at the point of the initial screen.

### How Should the Screening Instrument Be Selected and Used?

It is essential that a screening instrument focus on items that predict the kinds of long-term problems that are to be prevented. Violence and other antisocial behaviors in adolescence and early adulthood are best predicted in childhood by aggressive and disruptive behavior problems. For this reason, we chose the 10-item authority acceptance scale of the Teacher Observation of Classroom Adaptation—Revised (TOCA-R; Werthamer-Larsson et al., 1991), which described aggressive, disruptive, and oppositional behaviors. Teachers are often burdened with forms to complete on their students, and 10 items provided a diversity of problem behaviors without being very lengthy compared to most rating instruments. This measure showed a reasonable correlation with more lengthy measures of conduct problems in subsequent years (Lochman & CPPRG, 1995; Racz et al., 2013). The items of the TOCA-R used for the Fast Track teacher screen are included in Figure 10.1.

## What Kind of Cutoff Score Should Be Used with the Screening Instrument?

In the Fast Track screening process, cutoff scores were relative, and depended on the screening data collected each year. Each year, we collected ratings from all of the kindergarten teachers in the school district and then identified children with the highest scores. Subsequently, we conducted analyses to determine whether there was a specific cutoff

| *Directions:* In the last 3 weeks, would you say the following statements were never, rarely, sometimes, often, very often, or almost always true of this child? | | | | | | |
|---|---|---|---|---|---|---|
| *Items* | *Never* | *Rarely* | *Sometimes* | *Often* | *Very Often* | *Almost Always* |
| 1. Is stubborn | 1 | 2 | 3 | 4 | 5 | 6 |
| 2. Breaks rules | 1 | 2 | 3 | 4 | 5 | 6 |
| 3. Harms others | 1 | 2 | 3 | 4 | 5 | 6 |
| 4. Breaks things | 1 | 2 | 3 | 4 | 5 | 6 |
| 5. Takes others property | 1 | 2 | 3 | 4 | 5 | 6 |
| 6. Fights | 1 | 2 | 3 | 4 | 5 | 6 |
| 7. Lies | 1 | 2 | 3 | 4 | 5 | 6 |
| 8. Is disobedient | 1 | 2 | 3 | 4 | 5 | 6 |
| 9. Teases classmates | 1 | 2 | 3 | 4 | 5 | 6 |
| 10. Yells at others | 1 | 2 | 3 | 4 | 5 | 6 |

**FIGURE 10.1.** Items from the TOCA-R used for the Fast Track teacher screen.

on the teacher screen score that identified children at highest risk for future antisocial behavior and violence. We found that the association between the kindergarten teacher screen score and future antisocial behavior depended upon risk factors at the community level. In general, the proportion of youth at risk for later antisocial behavior and violent activity varied as a function of factors such as the level of neighborhood poverty and crime. Severity of child behavioral risk at kindergarten is one important risk factor, but neighborhood risks are also potent. Correspondingly, we believe that there is no single screen score cutoff that can identify youth at absolute risk; rather, the proportion and number of youth that a school or community needs to serve in a violence prevention program such as Fast Track will vary depending on neighborhood/community risk factors.

Arrests and incarceration result in high costs to a community, and we suggest that the rate of youth arrests can usefully serve as a general index of community-level risk and a base rate for change. As a result, we recommend that this percentage could serve as a rough indication of the cutoff score to be used with an instrument such as the TOCA-R for inclusion in the prevention program. Thus, communities with relatively high rates of adolescent violence and crime should offer prevention services to a greater proportion of youth than communities with lower base rates of juvenile crime. Whether the same cutoff score should be used for boys and girls is another issue that will come up in deciding who to include in the prevention program. The dilemma here is that while the percentage of girls showing problem behavior in the early school years will be lower than for boys in most communities, the subsequent rates of arrest in adolescence will be even lower for females than males, particularly for violent crimes. This may result in more "false positives" for girls than for boys if the goal is to reduce violence and crime, rather than substance abuse or early sexual activity, for example. In general, our recommendation is to use the same cutoff for boys and girls, but this decision will depend upon the local goals for prevention.

## Should the Screen Be Ongoing?

If the prevention program is meant to continue with the initially selected group of children beyond the first year of intervention, should the screening procedure be repeated on an ongoing basis? Our assumption is that for the program to have long-term effectiveness it should be viewed as a long-term process that prepares high-risk children with the skills and experiences they will need as they transition into school and life situations that challenge their vulnerabilities to become engaged in antisocial behaviors. Hence, the Fast Track model includes prevention services that extend across multiple years. In the Fast Track study, all children who were recruited initially into the program remained eligible for extended participation in the program, although the intensity of services they received varied as a function of the severity of their ongoing adjustment problems. However, this model is unlikely to work well in community settings for two reasons. First, as families move and children change schools, it may become impractical or unfeasible to serve them. Communities and schools will want to allow newly screened and recruited children to fill openings in the program left by families who leave. In addition, our data suggest that it was appropriate to reduce prevention services to children and families who showed improved competencies and reduced risk over time. Fast Track did not include a mechanism whereby children and families could graduate from the program based upon their progress, but our findings suggest that "early graduation" would have been a good idea for some children. In other words, we recommend using an ongoing assessment and screening process in order to allow for children and families to graduate out of the prevention program as they improve and in order to allow other children and families to enter the program based on their need (e.g., changing circumstances such as family or other trauma experiences or life stresses). Ongoing screening would also allow new children to enter the program and receive services. These children could be those we would consider "late starters" who did not have earlier conduct problems, as well as children who may have moved into the school who have had continuing difficulties.

## PROGRAM COMPONENTS AND STAFFING ARRANGEMENTS

As noted in earlier chapters, the original Fast Track elementary school program included seven components: the PATHS classroom curriculum, Parent Groups, home visiting, child social skill training groups (Friendship Groups), peer pairing, mentoring, and academic tutoring. Program delivery was provided by teams of FCs and ECs. The FCs were women, most with some college education and professional experience in assisting families, and the ECs were college-educated and experienced teachers, comfortable in assisting and consulting with teachers in the school setting and comfortable working with children who had behavior problems. FCs and ECs worked in pairs based on the cases in their charge and shared office space when not in the field. This arrangement worked well for Fast Track in the four different community settings where the program was implemented. These two different types of staff enabled us to schedule Parent and Friendship Group sessions simultaneously and permitted program staff to exchange information about the status of the family and their work with parents and children.

Since that time, the Fast Track model has now been implemented in a wide array of school districts and communities. In some cases, limited resources have required schools to make changes in program design in order to reduce the number of staff members needed to implement the program and to reduce associated costs. In this section, we describe the streamlined implementation models that best retain the core features of the Fast Track intervention model while reducing staff and implementation costs.

## Group versus Individualized Program Delivery

Conducting parent training in small groups has both advantages and disadvantages. The positive aspect of providing the training in groups is the shared interest and positive support that parents offer each other in the group. Parents in a group can exchange experiences relating to the group topic and thus broaden the framework of other members and, potentially, form the basis for parents supporting each other across time. Financial limitations also played a role in choosing to work in groups, as is often the case in prevention programs, because more families can be helped by fewer staff members. In addition, we felt that offering group sessions at the school may have helped us "market" the program to parents as well as to build positive school–family partnerships. When inviting parents into Fast Track, we described the program as a school enrichment program that included free reading tutoring, child friendship activities, and parent discussion groups focused on promoting the child's school success. We felt that this strengths-based approach was more appealing to parents than an alternative that focused on the child's behavior problems or school difficulties. Later in the program, when parents were interviewed about parts of the program they valued most and least, reading tutoring was generally valued most by parents and parent training groups were valued less so, but still valued. For this reason, we felt that the group structure of the original Fast Track program may have enhanced recruitment into the program.

We also implemented an individualized home-visiting approach to allow staff members to focus on parenting needs of each family and to adjust the pace and focus of support efforts to target specific skills and issues the parents needed. In addition, some parents were unable to attend a group or missed occasional sessions. Similarly, the decision to work with high-risk children in small groups was influenced heavily by practical factors. It seemed cost-effective to treat children in groups. In addition, groups provide children with opportunities to practice the social and self-control skills that were being taught in these groups and to do so under the observation of staff. On the other hand, conduct problem behaviors can be contagious and can serve to increase the overall disruptiveness of the group atmosphere. Some of our Friendship Groups, in fact, did contain too many seriously disruptive children, and this required a variety of strategies to provide a better learning environment, such as dividing children into smaller subgroups or including some well-functioning children in the groups.

An alternative strategy to conducting groups with high-risk children might have been to deliver skill-training content in the context of the peer-pairing sessions that were held in the school, rather than in the extracurricular groups. Peer-pairing sessions included a high-risk child and more socially skilled same-sex peer partners, who rotated over the course of the year. In our case, the decision to conduct child Friendship Groups was linked to the plan to have Parent Groups. Parents were attracted to attend these groups initially, in part, because reading tutoring was delivered after the Parent and Friendship Groups in first grade, and parents had the opportunity to observe a trained reading tutor work with their own child for a half hour each week. As noted below, in subsequent implementations of the Fast Track program, some schools and communities made changes in the administration of the Parent Groups and Friendship Groups, using alternative implementation arrangements to improve the feasibility and reduce the costs of the intervention.

### Adapting and Condensing the Child-Focused Programs

In the original program, staffing for the child-focused program components included an EC and a paraprofessional tutor. The EC ran the Friendship Group, coached classroom teachers in the use of the PATHS curriculum, and supervised the paraprofessional tutors. The tutors provided each child with three half-hour sessions per week (two tutoring sessions per week, one peer-pairing session). In first grade, tutors gave a third reading session in conjunction with the parenting and child groups, thus enabling parents to observe their child working with the tutor. In subsequent implementations of the Fast Track program, a number of school districts opted to drop the tutoring component from the Fast Track model and to eliminate the paraprofessional staff position. These school districts typically had other existing programs designed to address delays in the emergent literacy skills of entering kindergarten children, including Title 1 and other early-reading support programs, and hence felt that the Fast Track tutoring services were redundant.

A second modification that was made less often by school districts, but further reduced the cost of the Fast Track program, involved the implementation of the child social skill training program during school hours, rather than after school or on the weekend. When implemented during the school day, Friendship Groups typically included one to two "target" aggressive children and two to three peer partners from their classroom. In this way, the in-school Friendship Group combined the social skill training group program with the key features of the original peer-pairing program. The Friendship Group manual (Bierman, Greenberg, et al., 2017) has been written so that it can be used in both ways.

## Adapting and Condensing the Parent-Focused Programs

In the original program, FCs led the Parent Groups and also conducted home visits with participating families. A core feature of Fast Track was the implementation of the Friendship Group and the Parent Group at the same time, during a weekly 2-hour after-school or weekend session. With children and parents both present, it was possible to run a parent–child sharing session after the two separate group sessions. However, the implementation of family group sessions during out-of-school time was one of the more expensive and demanding features of the Fast Track model. Costs associated with these family sessions include transportation for the families, refreshments for parents and children, the provision of free child care, and payment to open the school building during non-school hours. It is not possible to determine what the long-term effects of Fast Track may have been had a more condensed implementation model been used, in which (1) only two staff positions were included (EC, FC); (2) tutoring was not provided; (3) Friendship Groups were combined with peer pairing and implemented during the school day; and (4) parent training was provided without accompanying transportation, food, and child care. Although these changes would substantially reduce the staff and budget demands associated with the Fast Track Program, while retaining the critical core elements of the PATHS curriculum in the classroom, child social skills training (Friendship Group), and parent education and support (Parent Group), it is not possible to determine just how much the impact of the program may be reduced. Support for group participation (e.g., transportation, child care, food, stipends) likely played a key role in sustaining attendance. In addition, Parent Groups and dyadic parent–child interaction experiences that were crafted during the Parent Groups are core features of the Fast Track intervention and could be responsible for intervention impact. Thus, it would be important to carefully assess the impact of this reduced program, preferably with an experimental design.

## Intensity of Services

It is also worth noting that these adaptations to the Fast Track implementation model also include differences in the scheduled intensity of the prevention services. In Fast Track, the intensity of intervention was massed in the beginning of the intervention and then tapered off in succeeding years. Parent and Friendship Groups met weekly in first grade, then every other week in the second grade, and monthly in succeeding years of elementary school. In deciding to taper off the frequency of the groups each succeeding year, we assumed that parents and children would assimilate most of the program content each year and be ready to build on it in succeeding years. However, the tapering down of the groups in this way is often not feasible given stable staffing patterns that characterize most school and community programs. In addition, the decision to hold groups once a month after second grade did not satisfy parents or staff. We originally conceptualized the monthly sessions as "booster" skill training and check-in systems. However, they did not seem to function in this way. In general, monthly groups were awkward for the staff, and were not frequent enough to sustain significant group cohesion or to support effective skill training. Hence, in retrospect, we would advise for a more even distribution of group sessions over the first 2 years of the program. We would also advise that, if the later-grade group sessions are used, these are massed in a set of booster sessions held weekly or biweekly for a shorter period of time, rather than scheduled monthly over a longer period of time.

## Engaging Parents and Teachers in the Intervention

In any prevention program, strategies to engage parents and teachers must be considered carefully. In particular, achieving high attendance rates at parenting sessions is always a challenge. This is a critically important issue because the success in reducing crime and violence in a community hinges on getting the intervention staff to recognize the importance of successfully engaging the highest-risk children and families into the preventive intervention. Intervention staff like to work with children and parents who are motivated to improve and are reliable in attending and participating in the program. In fact, some community-based mental health programs explicitly screen out unenthusiastic families, based on the assumption that they can only help the families who are enthusiastically engaged in intervention. This assumption fails to recognize that the degree of parent enthusiasm and engagement is often a direct result of the way in which program staff approach and encourage them to participate and the way in which the program is structured to reduce barriers to participation. Further, it is important to recognize that a substantial number of parents have been traumatized themselves, and it may take numerous attempts to solicit their participation. However, consider the long-term consequences of permitting as much as a third of the group screened for the intervention to be missing from the actual intervention due to poor recruitment approaches (and it is not unusual for prevention projects such as Fast Track to have an initial attrition level of 30%). This missing third may well contain that proportion of children who commit the most crimes in adolescence and would be the most violent through their life course. Parental neglect or inattention to children's needs is a major factor in the development of antisocial behavior. Failing to engage these families initially in the intervention is likely to defeat much of the purpose for starting the intervention in the first place.

This is an issue that is often not raised with staff in the initial training orientation but should be an important point of emphasis. At the outset of the Fast Track program, staff were told to approach families in a way that did not make initial participation an all-or-nothing proposition. The initial contacts were intended to build relationships. A similar perspective should be used in initial contacts with teachers, particularly in the implementation of PATHS, as noted earlier. An early focus on building relationships is likely to enhance parent and teacher participation and positive response over time. A rigid requirement of early adherence to program expectations may discourage some parents and teachers from participating, to the detriment of the children involved.

In Fast Track, we debated at length before starting the project whether additional incentives should be offered in order to improve parent participation. In addition to providing free transportation, child care, and refreshments at group sessions, we also offered parents a small cash incentive to attend the parenting sessions. Fast Track participants were mostly low-income families with limited financial opportunities; like the teachers, we justified paying them for their attendance as professional development funding, noting that by increasing their knowledge regarding how best to support their children's development, they would be costaff with us in our joint efforts to enhance their children's successful future. We did not approach parents with the message that their children were selected as at risk, as we believed that a focus on child risk and skill deficits would be perceived as judgmental and off-putting. As we have disseminated Fast Track, we have found that many schools and community agencies are unable or unwilling to offer families financial incentives for group participation. Without incentives, parent participation tends to be lower than when incentives are offered. For this reason, we encourage program administrators to consider alternative incentives very carefully, such as door prizes or gift certificates, as we believe that tangible incentives are quite important in creating the high attendance rates we experienced in Fast Track. Once families have established positive working relationships with program staff, the financial incentives become less important, as relationships with program staff and with other parents and the programming itself keep parents coming back.

An important fact emerged in the process of working with families. The overwhelming majority of parents, particularly mothers, were eager to have their children be as well-prepared for school and future success in life as possible. The hope for a positive school start and successful school experience appears to be fairly universal, despite concerns and fears in some cases that this will be hard to obtain. Although outside observers and school staff may find fault with the parenting experienced by many of the children who exhibit high rates of aggression, it should be recognized that most of these parents are parenting the way they were parented, and it takes time for them to recognize that they may need to learn some new ways. They do, however, recognize that their children may need help with academics and friendships, and this is why the services provided directly to the children were often the enticement for program participation.

Similarly, the receptiveness of teachers to including PATHS in the regular curriculum varied greatly. Some teachers embraced it quickly and used it effectively. Others resisted it in various ways or were stilted and ineffective in presenting it to children initially. Fast Track paid teachers to attend the PATHS workshop training and to attend consultation sessions with ECs, which occurred in addition to their regularly contracted work. We also had ECs spend time in the classroom with teachers at the beginning of the program, providing coteaching and classroom support to teachers. The capacity to offer these kinds of supports to teachers may vary depending upon the financial resources available to the program, but our sense is that they were quite important in terms of gaining a high level of teacher engagement in PATHS and supporting high-quality PATHS implementation.

## Alternative Staffing Models

In Fast Track, all staff were hired by the program, rather than working for the school district or a community agency. In some of the subsequent Fast Track implementations, the staffing plan has involved a partnership between a school district and a community agency. In these cases, FC staff members were hired by the community mental health agency to work with parents, and the EC staff were hired by a school district to work with children. Although this model can work, we found that it requires a level of coordination and communication between sponsoring agencies that can sometimes be difficult to attain and sustain. Arrangements for team building and communication within staff teams are needed, as well as the assurance of coordination and cooperation at the level of agency administrations. The adoption of this arrangement is predicated on the agreement by both agencies on the way financial costs will be handled, as well as ownership issues involving the staff.

Although it was never tried with Fast Track to our knowledge, an alternative arrangement used in some prevention programs is to have a single staff member handle the work of both the EC and FC. Obviously, each staff member would have to have a broad base of prior experience to cover these diverse intervention services. This alternative would likely work better if the training and case work were conducted with individual parents (and children) rather than in groups. Having a single staff person handle each case would eliminate the need for interagency collaboration, which certainly has its advantages. On the other hand, it might be difficult to find staff who would be credible to teachers and comfortable working with them in the classroom setting, as well as comfortable doing home visits with parents in less-than-stable family contexts, and running Friendship Groups (given the likely reduced effectiveness of a one-on-one approach with young children).

## Adolescent Programming

In the Fast Track program design, high-risk children and their families were identified at school entry and then followed longitudinally through their transition into middle and high school. This design made sense from the standpoint of the developmental model, but created some significant obstacles to efficient and effective prevention programming during the preadolescent and adolescent years. By the time of the middle school transition, there was considerable family mobility and geographical dispersion. For example, by grade 7, 25% of the intervention sample was no longer available to receive intervention services, primarily as a function of family moves outside of the possible service catchment area. By grade 10, 32% of the intervention sample was unavailable for intervention services. In addition, selecting children as at risk in kindergarten resulted in considerable heterogeneity in the risk status of the targeted youth by the time they reached early adolescence. As noted in Chapter 6, triannual assessments were conducted each year to characterize the nature and severity of adolescent risks. Across the domains rated (academic adjustment, peer relations, adult involvement, identity development), about one-third of the youth were rated in the minimal-risk range. These youth had recovered from their risky status in elementary school; had we screened for inclusion in adolescence, they would not have been selected. At the other end of the spectrum, about 20% of the sample were rated as demonstrating severe risk across several domains, indicating a need for intensive intervention. These youth had already become entrenched in significant levels of antisocial activity and dysfunctional adaptation. Had we not been constrained by the focused Fast Track model, we likely would have organized prevention services quite differently during the adolescent phase and we recommend that communities consider alternatives.

In Fast Track, we discontinued the provision of universal school-based services after children transitioned into middle school. In part this was necessary because students from intervention and control groups often entered the same middle schools. However, it was very difficult to support youth at school without the lever of an organized set of relationships with classroom teachers and school personnel parallel to that created during the elementary school years with the universal implementation of the PATHS curriculum. Once Fast Track children left elementary school, the task of trying to affect the classroom in ways that would enhance children's prosocial development became very difficult to achieve, given the need to rely on individual consultations with multiple teachers, without an overarching approach to unite these efforts. Effective universal prevention programs have been designed and tested with positive effects for the middle school and high school context (see reviews by Domitrovich, Syvertsen, & Calin, 2017; Lösel & Beelmann, 2003; Wilson & Lipsey, 2007). The advantages provided by a strong, evidence-based universal prevention program noted for the elementary school years also hold for the middle and high school years. Hence, whenever possible, we recommend that communities and schools invest in evidence-based universal prevention programming across the secondary school years.

It is also likely that communities and schools would benefit from rescreening youth at risk after the middle school transition, to better match youth and their families with the intensity of intervention services needed based upon their adolescent risk and protective factors. Based on the long-term data from Fast Track, it appears somewhat doubtful that the extended prevention supports provided to youth who were rated as minimal risk by the early adolescent years were needed or useful. On the other hand, youth who were rated as severe risk may have benefitted from more intensive, evidence-based treatments during adolescence, such as Multisystemic Therapy (Henggeler, 2011) or other evidence-based models (see reviews by Lösel & Beelmann, 2003; McMahon & Frick, 2019; Wilson & Lipsey, 2007).

Fast Track included a number of individualized services, based upon the developmental model. For example, when youth entered middle school, program content was developed to help Fast Track youth manage the challenges of dealing with peer pressure and the emerging risks for substance use, and to focus on their future vocational and career goals. As described in Chapter 6, these included four workshop sessions based on the school-to-jobs intervention (Oyserman et al., 2002) aimed at strengthening emerging identity and building a strong sense of future possibilities and goals (personal selves), and additional workshops that addressed vocational opportunities, life skills, and summer employment opportunities. A key goal of these sessions was to help youth identify the ways that they would like to see themselves as young adults and to clarify intermediate goals and tasks that would help them reach these longer-term goals. In this same vein, contacts were made with people in community workplaces of potential interest to individual youth, so that these youth might have experience in those workplaces and interview adults in their work roles. The YC organized these services. Often this YC was the same individual who had worked with a given child in the EC or FC role. However, because many of our ECs and ECs were women in their 30s and 40s, we attempted to recruit younger males as YCs for our male youth in order to provide them with role models who could relate more naturally with teens. Adult mentors were also sought to provide a separate source of guidance and influence beginning when children were in fourth grade. Often these mentors had a lengthy and influential role, but as successive cohorts of Fast Track youth became eligible for mentoring, it became more difficult to find mentors for the youth who most needed them, and with succeeding cohorts, our YCs tried to take on more of this role. Overall, these efforts to build youth hopes regarding their productive futures and provide support in moving toward those goals seemed worthwhile. However, future research is needed to understand how best to organize these kinds of prevention activities for maximal benefit.

## THE BIG PICTURE: COMMUNITY PLANNING AND PREVENTION

The discussion thus far has focused on school and family-involved programs and staff interactions that build parenting skills that will promote a supportive home and nurture the child's own self-regulation skills, finding nonaggressive solutions to frustrating situations with peers and teachers, and avoiding negative peer pressure. All of this early programming sets the stage for transitions into adolescence and young adulthood that take youth closer to the goals they have developed for themselves. At this point, it is imperative that a community that seeks to reduce youth antisocial behavior and violence must also provide resources and opportunities for youth to realize work and relational goals in ways that, in turn, help them to feel supported by and bond with the community.

## School and Community Contextual Factors

The larger context of community support for reducing risk for violence is important at all phases of the developmental process. Initially, there are homes and classrooms that unwittingly promote conduct problems. In every community, there are families that are formed by parents whose own backgrounds leave them unprepared for parenting. When these parents raise their children in more violence-prone neighborhoods, the probability of their children becoming more aggressive increases greatly. This is one of the ways in which community context makes a difference.

Many of the Fast Track children attended schools that had high levels of conduct problems, as well as low levels of academic achievement. This context usually matched the neighborhoods in which they lived. As an example, while making a home visit, one of our staff was told by a passing police officer that they, the police, only came to that neighborhood in pairs and in vehicles. The challenge for us in the Fast Track project was to help children overcome the deleterious influences of the contexts in which they were growing up, including deeply engrained institutional racism and classism that many parents and youth experienced on a daily basis. In the most difficult of circumstances this proved to be more of a challenge than we could meet, even with experienced and dedicated intervention staff. For example, some Fast Track children, boys particularly, were recruited at a very young age to be "runners" for drug sales in the neighborhood. In some cases, Fast Track children had older siblings who simply brought them into the game at an early age, sometimes with the tacit consent of their parents.

Social services in most communities do their best to help parents with these issues, but they are often limited in the time and resources that they can commit. Other agencies may also aid in this process, but often there is a lack of coordination in these interagency efforts and they rarely have time for prevention efforts, as their time and resources are focused on dealing with children and families currently in crisis. Once children enter school, and for much of childhood, the school becomes the community agency that bears the heaviest responsibility for the socialization of at-risk children and the provision of prevention-oriented programming. Teachers who face classrooms that contain many children with risk for conduct problems have a far greater challenge to their effectiveness than do teachers with only a few such children in their class. Some teachers are better prepared to work with these children than others, but even the best teachers are ill-prepared to deal with a classroom that has as many as seven or eight children exhibiting high rates of challenging behavior. In these kinds of classrooms, at-risk children are more likely to form bonds with other aggressive children in ways that escalate their aggression and increase their risk for future antisocial activity.

## Interface with Juvenile Justice

By the time that a youth commits violent acts, it becomes the job of police and judicial authorities to intervene. The contentious interaction between adolescents and police is an issue that has become a topic of greater focus currently, particularly in neighborhoods comprised of families of color. Our experience in relating to parents on this issue was framed by our black staff members, who recounted the importance of "the talk" that most of them received as early adolescents. This phenomenon is receiving more general discussion in the press these days, but it involves warning black youth of the personal safety issues in their reactions to police contact, as well as augmenting their understanding of stereotyping minority teens and the history of institutional racism. We did not reach out to police departments to try to develop sensitivity to this issue from their side of the interaction, however. This goal is something that probably requires careful interagency communication and timing. Sometimes neighborhood watch and youth recreation programs are promoted in the service of prevention. Social services most often take the role of helping parents of children with conduct problems but are limited in what they can do to help them in developing prosocial skills in their children.

It is essential that communities look at the bigger picture and realize that in both highly urban and poor rural communities, children growing up in neighborhoods of concentrated disadvantage witness the reality that incarceration is a common life event among family and community members. The "prison boom" of the past two decades has considerably deepened the intergenerational experience of children, many of whom have compromised mental health and cognitive impairment and are likely to engage in violence. Thus, creating the support systems and building the protective factors necessary for the success of the next generation requires "rethinking" the problem and having a reengineered solution that demands a new level of multistakeholder community engagement.

## Fostering Collective Action

Our sense is that to successfully develop and sustain comprehensive programs such as Fast Track requires collective action, often termed "collective impact," that requires the involvement of a variety of community partners/stakeholders. These partners include not only schools, families, and mental health service agencies, but also agencies attempting to prevent drug abuse and juvenile delinquency (police, judges, probation), and community-level charities such as the United Way and the business community. To carry out such comprehensive and long-term models requires a community-level prevention infrastructure that can champion the needs of children and their families who often lack representation.

Often there are multiple agencies that take on some level of responsibility to reduce juvenile violence and crime, but finding ways to communicate and coordinate efforts across these different agencies is often a challenge. Sustaining efforts over time is also difficult. For example, although Fast Track began with the consent and support of school district superintendents, school principals, and classroom teachers, programs such as Fast Track do not sustain themselves across time without the continuing long-term support of these individuals, and of those who follow them in these positions. School superintendents, for example, change jobs every 3 or 4 years (Grissom & Anderson, 2012). More than 70% of superintendents from large urban districts leave within 3 years and thus often have little stake in investing in the "long game" of comprehensive models. Given the high rate of transition, even if a superintendent implements such a vision, the desire for program or policy "ownership" can mean that programs started under one administration can lose support under a new leader. This ownership issue holds at every level—district, school, and classroom—but it is particularly relevant at the level of school's district superintendent.

To facilitate the goals of coordinated and sustained community efforts, prevention program ownership is ideally shared among multiple community leaders so that both financial support and program continuity are maintained across the time necessary to have meaningful impact. There are a number of examples of potential models that create collective action involving multiple stakeholders making long-term commitments. For example, Communities That Care is a broad community-based model for supporting youth development and reducing violence, aggression, and crime (Kim, Gloppen, Rhew, Oesterle, & Hawkins, 2015). A second approach is the StriveTogether model of collective efficacy that began in Cincinnati and that attempts collective action at the level of a long-term community partnership to improve the well-being and educational outcomes of children (*www.strivetogether.org*). A third example is the PROSPER model, which links university experts with school–community teams to facilitate the implementation of school-based and family-focused evidence-based programming (*www.blueprintsprograms.com/factsheet/prosper*). The adage, "It takes a village to raise a child" is easy to say but extremely hard to maintain in practice. These are all examples of effective comprehensive community initiatives (*www. americaspromise.org/resource/promise-comprehensive-community-initiatives*). It is easier to start a prevention program in a community that has a single strong leader who supports it, but it is harder to sustain that program when that leader moves on. For this reason, we urge those wanting to emulate a program like Fast Track in their community to spend the time necessary to build consensus among community leaders.

## How Might Such a Community Consensus Be Built?

This part of our discussion is even more speculative because it is hard to point to examples that have been sustained for as long a period of time as the Fast Track program required. Fast Track was started and funded for a planned length of time and when that funding ended, the program also ended, or at best, program components were kept going on a limited basis. In that light, it must be said that we failed in ways that we are encouraging communities not to replicate.

We have articulated our sense of the reason why single-owner programs dissipate. We have suggested that community ownership is essential for long-term sustainability and that it is difficult to establish at the outset without sufficient buy-in by leaders across sectors. Although funding is very often a major obstacle, there are other obstacles. Building community consensus, at some level, is the starting point. Concerned individuals, who might be school board members or administrators, city or county board members, clergy, members of the judiciary or policing units, social service administrators, or local foundation officers or board members are the most logical people to reach out to others to discuss solutions to violence and serious crime in their community. Such discussions could lead to the type of comprehensive planning needed to adopt a program having some features similar to Fast Track. In our view, the participation of school administrators and school board members in such planning is critical, but schools cannot be left to shoulder the principal burdens of staffing and funding.

If there is consensus among a critical mass of the stakeholders that a comprehensive prevention program should be initiated, clear responsibility needs to be established for the various tasks that delineate fiduciary, administrative, and programming roles as well as all the work roles that funding, staffing, and training will entail. From the outset, it is necessary to recognize that stakeholders will change roles (job changes, moves, retirements, etc.) and thus to sustain such efforts means having a very clear organization structure, mission, and goals as well as procedures for onboarding new coalition members. Although an inspirational and visible key leader is often necessary to launch multi-agency initiatives, sustainability requires clear organizational structure and ongoing community outreach. Important areas of focus include adequate early training of key leaders so that they are knowledgeable and have a high degree of competence in understanding the long-term investment and logic model that underlies the prevention program's purpose, efforts, and actions (Feinberg, Greenberg, & Osgood, 2004). Ongoing high-quality technical assistance that helps the coalition/board maintain fidelity to the model and creates effective internal board functioning (e.g., high cohesion, task orientation, and performance) is also essential. In addition, clearly establishing benchmarks for program success and assessing them on a periodic level can provide the types of data that encourage program continuation. The challenge of maintaining sufficient community support and funding for such long-term efforts is tremendous, requiring substantial planning, resources, and skill.

## SUMMARY

In most communities, there exists a level of violence and serious crime that is of substantial community concern. The dramatic long-term success of Fast Track in reducing these levels of violence and serious crime can provide an outline for the critical features of a prevention effort. Here, we have focused on how key program components of Fast Track may be implemented in various ways depending on funding and other community considerations.

We advise that screening of high-risk individuals be done prior to the end of the first year of organized schooling (usually kindergarten), when development of these problems is sufficiently stable for accurate prediction to longer-term problems but while change in behavior can be diverted from a long-term path of antisocial behavior. Screening levels should be set according to base rates of youth and young adult arrest and conviction rates, usually by gender. Screening should probably be ongoing in order to include later starters and to discontinue services to those who no longer seem to need them. Variations in staffing for particular community and agency resources and function are outlined, and this is where a community-level advisory coalition or board may be both useful and necessary. A proactive community coalition that includes essential community leaders and stakeholders can assure both continuity of effort and strategy while making needed changes in direction that occur as communities evolve.

## A FINAL NOTE

At the beginning of this volume we expressed our gratitude to federal agencies, particularly NIMH, for the substantial financial support and vision that made this venture possible. Our hope when we launched the program was that the results of this complex prevention trial would provide guidance to communities and community leaders in their efforts to prevent violence and crime, as well as psychiatric disorders, in their communities. This continues to be our hope even though the times in which we live are now different.

Three decades ago our nation was in the midst of a serious upsurge in violent crime and our nation's leaders initiated and sustained a commitment to finding an answer to this upsurge. At the point of this writing, there is still significant violence and crime in our communities, but our national focus is more diffuse and uncertain. This will, no doubt, make it harder to replicate what FastTrack has accomplished, but we hope that the publication of this volume will stimulate conversations in communities everywhere about the feasibility of protecting their community and their youth from the kinds of behavior that stimulated our efforts years ago.

# References

Achenbach, T. M. (1991a). *Manual for the Child Behavior Checklist 4–18 and 1991 Profile*. Burlington: University of Vermont Department of Psychiatry.

Achenbach, T. M. (1991b). *Manual for the Teacher's Report Form*. Burlington: University of Vermont, Department of Psychiatry.

Albert, D., Belsky, D. W., Crowley, D. M., Bates, J. E., Pettit, G. S., Lansford, J. E., . . . Dodge, K. A. (2015). Developmental mediation of genetic variation in response to the Fast Track prevention program. *Development and Psychopathology, 27,* 81–95.

Albert, D., Belsky, D. W., Crowley, D. M., Latendresse, S. J., Aliev, F., Riley, B., . . . Dodge, K. A. (2015). Can genetics predict response to complex behavioral interventions?: Evidence from a genetic analysis of the Fast Track randomized control trial. *Journal of Policy Analysis and Management, 34,* 497–518.

Anton, M. T., & Jones, D. J. (2017). Adoption of technology-enhanced treatments: Conceptual and practice considerations. *Clinical Psychology: Science and Practice, 24,* 223–240.

Arnold, M. E., & Hughes, J. N. (1999). First do no harm: Adverse effects of grouping deviant youth for skills training. *Journal of School Psychology, 37,* 99–115.

Asarnow, J. (l983). Children with peer adjustment problems: Sequential and nonsequential analyses of school behaviors. *Journal of Consulting and Clinical Psychology, 51,* 709–717.

Battistich, V., Schaps, E., Watson, M., & Solomon, D. (1996). Prevention effects of the Child Development Project: Early findings from an ongoing multisite demonstration trial. *Journal of Adolescent Research, 11,* 12–35.

Battistich, V., Solomon, D., Watson, M., Solomon, J., & Schaps, E. (1989). Effects of an elementary school program to enhance prosocial behavior on children's cognitive social problem-solving skills and strategies. *Journal of Applied Developmental Psychology, 10,* 147–169.

Baydar, N., Reid, M. J., & Webster-Stratton, C. (2003). The role of mental health factors and program engagement in the effectiveness of a preventive parenting program for Head Start mothers. *Child Development, 74,* 1433–1453.

Bennett, K. J., Lipman, E. L., Brown, S., Racine, Y., Boyle, M. H., & Offord, D. R. (1999). Predicting conduct problems: Can high-risk children be identified in kindergarten and grade 1? *Journal of Consulting and Clinical Psychology, 67,* 470–480.

Bennett, K. J., & Offord, D. R. (2001). Screening for conduct disorder: Does the predictive accuracy of conduct disorder symptoms improve with age? *Journal of the American Academy of Child and Adolescent Psychiatry, 40,* 1418–1425.

Bierman, K. L. (1986). Process of change during social skills training with preadolescents and its relation to treatment outcome. *Child Development, 57,* 230–240.

Bierman, K. L. (2004). *Peer rejection: Developmental processes and intervention strategies.* New York: Guilford Press.

Bierman, K. L., Bruschi, C., Domitrovich, C., Fang, G. Y., Miller-Johnson, S., & Conduct Problems Prevention Research Group (CPPRG). (2004). Early disruptive behaviors associated with emerging antisocial behavior among girls. In M. Putallaz & K. L. Bierman (Eds.), *Aggression, antisocial behavior, and violence among girls: A developmental perspective* (pp. 137–161). New York: Guilford Press.

Bierman, K. L., & Furman, W. (1984). The effects of social skills training and peer involvement on the social adjustment of preadolescents. *Child Development, 55,* 151–162.

Bierman, K. L., Greenberg, M. T., Coie, J. D., Dodge, K. A., Lochman, J. E., & McMahon, R. J. (2017). *Social and emotional skills training for children: The Fast Track Friendship Group manual.* New York: Guilford Press.

Bierman, K. L., Greenberg, M. T., & Conduct Problems Prevention Research Group. (1996). Social skill training in the Fast Track program. In R. D. Peters & R. J. McMahon (Eds.), *Preventing childhood disorders, substance abuse, and delinquency* (pp. 65–89). Newbury Park, CA: SAGE.

Bierman, K. L., Heinrichs, B. S., Welsh, J. A., Nix, R. L., & Gest, S. D. (2017). Enriching preschool classrooms and home visits with evidence-based programming: Sustained benefits for low-income children. *Journal of Child Psychology and Psychiatry, 58,* 129–137.

Bierman, K. L., Nix, R. L., Maples, J. J., Murphy, S. A., & Conduct Problems Prevention Research Group. (2006). Examining the use of clinical judgment in the context of an adaptive prevention design: The Fast Track program. *Journal of Consulting and Clinical Psychology, 74,* 468–481.

Bierman, K. L., & Powers, C. J. (2009). Social skills training to improve peer relations. In K. H. Rubin, W. Bukowski, & B. Laursen (Eds.), *Handbook of peer interactions, relationships, and groups* (pp. 603–621). New York: Guilford Press.

Bierman, K. L., & Torres, M. (2016). Promoting the development of executive functions through early education and prevention programs. In J. A. Griffin, L. S. Freund, & P. McCardle (Eds.), *Executive function in preschool age children: Integrating measurement, neurodevelopment and translational research* (pp. 299–326). Washington, DC: American Psychological Association.

Bishop, D., Bryant, K. S., Giles, S. M., Hansen, W. B., & Dusenbury, L. (2006). Simplifying the delivery of a prevention program with web-based enhancements. *Journal of Primary Prevention, 27,* 433–444.

Black, E., Panzer, R. J., Mayewski, R. J., & Griner, P. F. (1991). Characteristics of diagnostic tests and principles for their use in quantitative decision making. In R. Panzer, E. R. Black, & P. F. Griner (Eds.), *Diagnostic strategies for common medical problems* (pp. 1–16). Washington, DC: American College of Physicians.

Blair, C., & Raver, C. C. (2015). School readiness and self-regulation: A developmental psychobiological approach. *Annual Review of Psychology, 66,* 711–731.

Blumstein, A. (1995). Youth violence, guns, and the illicit-drug industry. *Journal of Criminal Law and Criminology, 86,* 10–36.

Blumstein, A., Cohen, J., Roth, J. A., & Visher, C. A. (1986). *Criminal careers and "career criminals."* Washington, DC: National Academy Press.

Bögels, S., Hoogstad, B., van Dun, L., de Schutter, S., & Restifo, K. (2008). Mindfulness training for adolescents with externalizing disorders and their parents. *Behavioural and Cognitive Psychotherapy, 36,* 193–209.

Bögels, S., & Restifo, K. (2014). *Mindful parenting.* New York: Springer.

Boisjoli, R., Vitaro, F., Lacourse, É., Barker, E. D., & Tremblay, R. E. (2007). Impact and clinical significance of a preventive intervention for disruptive boys: 15-year follow-up. *British Journal of Psychiatry, 191,* 415–419.

Boivin, M., Dodge, K. A., & Coie, J. D. (1995). Individual-group behavioral similarity and peer status in experimental play groups of boys: The social misfit revisited. *Journal of Personality and Social Psychology, 69,* 269–279.

Botvin, G. (1986). Substance abuse prevention efforts: Recent developments and future directions. *Journal of School Health, 56,* 369–374.

Boxmeyer, C. L., Lochman, J. E., Powell, N. R., Windle, M., & Wells, K. (2008). School counselors' implementation of Coping Power in a dissemination field trial: Delineating the range of flexibility within fidelity. *Report on Emotional and Behavioral Disorders in Youth, 8,* 79–95.

Boyce, W. T., & Ellis, B. J. (2005). Biological sensitivity to context: I. An evolutionary-developmental theory of the origins and functions of stress reactivity. *Development and Psychopathology, 17,* 271–301.

Boyd-Ball, A., & Dishion, T. J. (2006). Family-centered treatment for American Indian adolescent substance abuse: Toward a culturally and historically informed strategy. In H. A. Liddle & C. L. Rowe (Eds.), *Adolescent substance abuse: Research and clinical advances* (pp. 423–448). New York: Cambridge University Press.

Breitenstein, S. M., Gross, D., & Christophersen, R. (2014). Digital delivery methods of parenting training interventions: A systematic review. *Worldviews on Evidence-Based Nursing, 11,* 168–176.

Brody, G. H., Beach, S. R. H., Hill, K. G., Howe, G. W., Prado, G., & Fullerton, S. M. (2013). Using genetically informed, randomized prevention trials to test etiological hypotheses about child and adolescent drug use and psychopathology. *American Journal of Public Health, 103,* S19–S24.

Bronfenbrenner, U. (1979). *The ecology of human development.* Cambridge, MA: Harvard University Press.

Brown, B. B., & Klute, C. (2003). Friendships, cliques, and crowds. In G. R. Adams & M. D. Berzonsky (Eds.), *Blackwell handbooks of developmental psychology. Blackwell handbook of adolescence* (pp. 330–348). Oxford, UK: Blackwell.

Brown, C. F. (1993). Statistical methods for preventive trials in mental health. *Statistics in Medicine, 12,* 289–300.

Cabot, R. C. (1931). Treatment in social case work and the need of criteria and tests of its success of failure. In *Proceedings of the National Conference on Social Welfare,* pp. 435–453.

Campbell, S. B. (2002). *Behavior problems in preschool children: Clinical and developmental issues* (2nd ed.). New York: Guilford Press.

Capaldi, D. M., Crosby, L., & Stoolmiller, M. (1996). Predicting the timing of first sexual intercourse for at-risk adolescent males. *Child Development, 67,* 344–359.

Carre, J. M., Iselin, A. M. R., Welker, K. M., Hariri, A. R., & Dodge, K. A. (2014). Testosterone reactivity to provocation mediates the effect of early intervention on aggressive behavior. *Psychological Science, 25,* 1140–1146.

Carsley, D., Khoury, B., & Heath, N. L. (2018). Effectiveness of mindfulness interventions for mental health in schools: A comprehensive meta-analysis. *Mindfulness, 9,* 693–707.

Caspi, A., Lynam, D., Moffitt, T. E., & Silva, P. (1993). Unraveling girls' delinquency: Biological, dispositional, and contextual contributions to adolescent misbehavior. *Developmental Psychology, 29,* 19–30.

Cernkovich, S. A., & Giordano, P. C. (2001). Stability and change in antisocial behaviour: The transition from adolescence to early adulthood. *Criminology, 39,* 371–410.

Chacko, A., Jensen, S. A., Lowry, L. S., Cornwell, M., Chimklis, A., Chan, E., . . . Pulgarin, B. (2016). Engagement in behavioral parent training: Review of the literature and implications for practice. *Clinical Child and Family Psychology Review, 19,* 204–215.

Chou, T., Bry, L. J., & Comer, J. S. (2017). Overcoming traditional barriers only to encounter new ones: Doses of caution and direction as technology-enhanced treatments begin to "go live." *Clinical Psychology: Science and Practice, 24,* 241–244.

Cicchetti, D., & Richters, J. E. (1993). Developmental considerations in the investigation of conduct disorder. *Development and Psychopathology, 5,* 331–344.

Cicchetti, D., & Toth, S. L. (1998). Perspectives on research and practice in developmental psychopathology. In W. Damon, I. E. Sigel, & K. A.

Renninger (Eds.), *Handbook of child psychology: Vol. 4. Child psychology in practice* (5th ed., pp. 479–583). Hoboken, NJ: Wiley.

Coatsworth, J. D., Duncan, L. D., Nix, R. L., Greenberg, M. T., Gayles, J. G., Bamberger, K. T., . . . Demi, M. A. (2015). Integrating mindfulness with parent training: Effects of the mindfulness-enhanced Strengthening Families Program. *Developmental Psychology, 51,* 26–35.

Cohen, M. A. (1988). Pain, suffering, and jury awards: A study of the cost of crime to victims. *Law and Society Review, 22,* 537–556.

Cohen, M., & Piquero, A. R. (2009). New evidence on the monetary value of saving a high risk youth. *Journal of Quantitative Criminology, 25,* 25–49.

Coie, J. D. (1990). Toward a theory of peer rejection. In S. R. Asher & J. D. Coie (Eds.), *Peer rejection in childhood* (pp. 365–401). New York: Cambridge University Press.

Coie, J. D., & Dodge, K. A. (1998). Aggression and antisocial behavior. In W. Damon (Ed.) & N. Eisenberg (Vol. Ed.), *Handbook of child psychology: Vol. 3. Social, emotional, and personality development* (pp. 779–861). New York: Wiley.

Coie, J. D., & Koeppl, G. K. (1990). Adapting intervention to the problems of aggressive and disruptive rejected children. In S. R. Asher & J. D. Coie (Eds.), *Peer rejection in childhood* (pp. 309–337). New York: Cambridge University Press.

Coie, J. D., & Krehbiel, G. (1984). Effects of academic tutoring on the social status of low-achieving, socially-rejected children. *Child Development, 55,* 1465–1478.

Coie, J. D., Lochman, J. E., Terry, R., & Hyman, C. (1992). Predicting early adolescent disorders from childhood aggression and peer rejection. *Journal of Consulting and Clinical Psychology, 60,* 783–792.

Coie, J. D., Watt, N. F., West, S. G., Hawkins, J. D., Asarnow, J. R., Markman, H. J., . . . Long, B. (1993). The science of prevention: A conceptual framework and some directions for a national research program. *American Psychologist, 48,* 1013–1022.

Cole, S. W. (2013). Social regulation of human gene expression: Mechanisms and implications for public health. *American Journal of Public Health, 103,* S84–S92.

Collins, L. M., Baker, T. B., Mermelstein, R. J., Piper, M. E., Jorenby, D. E., Smith, S. S., . . . Fiore, M. C. (2011). The Multiphase Optimization Strategy for engineering effective tobacco use interventions. *Annals of Behavioral Medicine, 41,* 208–226.

Collins, L. M., Murphy, S. A., & Bierman, K. L. (2004). A conceptual framework for adaptive preventive interventions. *Prevention Science, 5,* 185–196.

Comer, J. S., Furr, J. M., Miguel, E. M., Cooper-Vince, C. E., Carpenter, A. L., Elkins, M., . . . Chase, R. (2017). Remotely delivering real-time parent training to the home: An initial randomized trial of Internet-delivered Parent–Child Interaction Therapy (I-PCIT). *Journal of Consulting and Clinical Psychology, 85,* 909–917.

Conduct Problems Prevention Research Group. (1992). A developmental and clinical model for the prevention of conduct disorders: The FAST Track program. *Development and Psychopathology, 4,* 509–528.

Conduct Problems Prevention Research Group. (1999a). Initial impact of the Fast Track prevention trial for conduct problems: I. The high-risk sample. *Journal of Consulting and Clinical Psychology, 67,* 631–647.

Conduct Problems Prevention Research Group. (1999b). Initial impact of the Fast Track prevention trial for conduct problems: II. Classroom effects. *Journal of Consulting and Clinical Psychology, 67,* 648–657.

Conduct Problems Prevention Research Group. (2000). Merging universal and indicated prevention programs: The Fast Track model. *Addictive Behaviors, 25,* 913–927.

Conduct Problems Prevention Research Group. (2002a). Evaluation of the first 3 years of the Fast Track prevention trial with children at high risk for adolescent conduct problems. *Journal of Abnormal Child Psychology, 30,* 19–35.

Conduct Problems Prevention Research Group. (2002b). Using the Fast Track randomized prevention trial to test the early-starter model of the development of serious conduct problems. *Development and Psychopathology, 14,* 925–943.

Conduct Problems Prevention Research Group. (2004a). The effects of the Fast Track program on serious problem outcomes at the end of elementary school. *Journal of Clinical Child and Adolescent Psychology, 33,* 650–661.

Conduct Problems Prevention Research Group. (2004b). The Fast Track experiment: Translating the developmental model into a prevention design. In J. B. Kupersmidt & K. A. Dodge (Eds.), *Children's peer relations: From development to intervention* (pp. 181–208). Washington, DC: American Psychological Association.

Conduct Problems Prevention Research Group. (2007). The Fast Track randomized controlled trial to prevent externalizing psychiatric disorders. *Journal of the American Academy of Child and Adolescent Psychiatry, 46,* 319–333.

Conduct Problems Prevention Research Group. (2010a). The difficulty of maintaining positive intervention effects: A look at disruptive behavior, deviant peer relations, and social skills during the middle school years. *Journal of Early Adolescence, 30,* 593–624.

Conduct Problems Prevention Research Group. (2010b). Fast Track intervention effects on youth arrests and delinquency. *Journal of Experimental Criminology, 6,* 131–157.

Conduct Problems Prevention Research Group. (2010c). The effects of a multi-year randomized clinical trial of a universal social-emotional learning program: The role of student and school characteristics. *Journal of Consulting and Clinical Psychology, 78,* 156–168.

Conduct Problems Prevention Research Group. (2011). The effects of the Fast Track preventive intervention on the development of conduct disorder across childhood. *Child Development, 82,* 331–345.

Conduct Problems Prevention Research Group. (2013). School outcomes of aggressive-disruptive children: Prediction from kindergarten risk factors and impact of the Fast Track prevention program. *Aggressive Behavior, 39,* 114–130.

Conduct Problems Prevention Research Group. (2014). Trajectories of risk for early sexual activity and early substance use in the Fast Track prevention program. *Prevention Science, 15*(Suppl. 1), S33–S46.

Conduct Problems Prevention Research Group. (2015). Impact of early intervention on psychopathology, crime, and well-being at age 25. *American Journal of Psychiatry, 172,* 59–70.

Connell, A., Dishion, T., Yasui, M., & Kavanagh, K. (2007). An adaptive approach to family intervention: Linking engagement in family-centered intervention to reductions in adolescent problem behavior. *Journal of Consulting and Clinical Psychology, 75,* 568–579.

Creswell, J. D., Way, B. M., Eisenberger, N. I., & Lieberman, M. D. (2007). Neural correlates of dispositional mindfulness during affect labeling. *Psychosomatic Medicine, 69,* 560–565.

Crockett, L. J., Raffaelli, M., & Shen, Y. (2006). Linking self-regulation and risk proneness to risky sexual behavior: Pathways through peer pressure and early substance use. *Journal of Research on Adolescence, 16,* 503–525.

Cuijpers, P. (2003). Examining the effects of prevention programs on the incidence of new cases of mental disorders: The lack of statistical power. *American Journal of Psychiatry, 160,* 1385–1391.

Dadds, M. R., Cauchi, A. J., Wimalaweera, S., Hawes, D. J., & Brennan, J. (2012). Outcomes, moderators, and mediators of empathic-emotion recognition training for complex conduct problems in childhood. *Psychiatry Research, 199,* 201–207.

Damon, W. (2008). *The path to purpose: How young people find their calling in life.* New York: Free Press.

Diamond, A., & Lee, K. (2011). Interventions shown to aid executive function development in children 4–12 years old. *Science, 333,* 959–964.

Dilulio, J. J. (1995, November 27). The coming of the super-predators. *The Weekly Standard.*

Dishion, T. J., & Andrews, D. W. (1995). Preventing escalation in problem behaviors with high-risk young adolescents: Immediate and 1-year outcomes. *Journal of Consulting and Clinical Psychology, 63,* 538–548.

Dishion, T. J., Dodge, K. A., & Lansford, J. E. (2006). Findings and recommendations: A blueprint to minimize deviant peer influence in youth interventions and programs. In K. A. Dodge, T. J. Dishion, & J. E. Lansford (Eds.), *Deviant peer influences in programs for youth: Problems and solutions* (pp. 366–394). New York: Guilford Press.

Dishion, T. J., McCord, J., & Poulin, F. (1999). When interventions harm: Peer groups and problem behavior. *American Psychologist, 54,* 755–764.

Dishion, T. J., Piehler, T. F., & Myers, M. W. (2008). Dynamics and ecology of adolescent peer influence. In M. J. Prinstein & K. A. Dodge (Eds.), *Understanding peer influence in children and adolescents* (pp. 72–93). New York: Guilford Press.

Dishion, T. J., Poulin, F., & Burraston, B. (2001). Peer group dynamics associated with iatrogenic effects in group interventions with high-risk young adolescents. In D. W. Nangle & C. A. Erdley (Eds.), *The role of friendship in psychological adjustment* (pp. 79–92). San Francisco: Jossey-Bass.

Dishion, T. J., & Stormshak, E. (2007). *Intervening in children's lives: An ecological, family-centered approach to mental health care.* Washington, DC: American Psychological Association.

Dishion, T. J., & Tipsord, J. M (2011). Peer contagion in adolescent social and emotional development. *Annual Review of Psychology, 62,* 189–214.

Dodge, K. A. (1993). The future of research on the treatment of conduct disorder. *Development and Psychopathology, 5,* 311–319.

Dodge, K. A., Bates, J. E., & Pettit, G. S. (1990). Mechanisms in the cycle of violence. *Science, 250,* 1678–1683.

Dodge, K. A., Coie, J. D., & Lynam, D. (2006). Aggression and antisocial behavior in youth. In N. Eisenberg, W. Damon, & R. M. Lerner (Eds.), *Handbook of child psychology: Vol. 3. Social, emotional, and personality development* (6th ed., pp. 719–788). Hoboken, NJ: Wiley.

Dodge, K. A., Godwin, J., & Conduct Problems Prevention Research Group. (2013). Social-information-processing patterns mediate the impact of preventive intervention on adolescent antisocial behavior. *Psychological Science, 24,* 456–465.

Dodge, K. A., Greenberg, M. T., Malone, P. S., & Conduct Problems Prevention Research Group. (2008). Testing an idealized dynamic cascade model of the development of serious violence in adolescence. *Child Development, 79,* 1907–1927.

Domitrovich, C. E., Syvertsen, A. K., & Calin, S. S. (2017). *Promoting social and emotional learning in the middle and high school years.* University Park: Edna Bennett Pierce Prevention Research Center, Pennsylvania State University.

Dubois, D., & Karcher, M. (Eds). (2006). *Handbook of youth mentoring.* Thousand Oaks, CA: SAGE.

Dumas, J. E. (2005). Mindfulness-based parent training: Strategies to lessen the grip of automaticity in families with disruptive children. *Journal of Clinical Child and Adolescent Psychology, 34,* 779–791.

Dumas, J. E., Nissley-Tsiopinis, J., & Moreland, A. D. (2007). From intent to enrollment, attendance, and participation in preventive parenting groups. *Journal of Child and Family Studies, 16,* 1–26.

Duncan, G. J., Ludwig, J., & Magnusson, K. A. (2007). Reducing poverty through preschool interventions. *The Future of Children, 17,* 143–160.

Duncan, L. J., Coatsworth, D. J., & Greenberg, M. T. (2009). A model of mindful parenting: Implications for parent–child relationships and prevention research. *Clinical Child and Family Psychology Review, 12,* 255–270.

Durlak, J. A., & DuPre, E. P. (2008). Implementation matters: A review of research on the influence of implementation on program outcomes and the factors affecting implementation. *American Journal of Community Psychology, 41,* 327–350.

Durlak, J. A., Weissberg, R. P., Dymnicki, A. B., Taylor, R. D., & Schellinger,

K. B. (2011). The impact of enhancing students' social and emotional learning: A meta-analysis of school-based universal interventions. *Child Development, 82,* 405–432.

Eccles, J. E., Midgley, C. M., & Adler, T. (1984). Age-related changes in the school environment: Effects on achievement motivation. In J. P. Nicholls (Ed.), *The development of achievement motivation* (pp. 283–331). Greenwich, CT: JAI Press.

Eddy, J. M., Reid, J. B., Stoolmiller, M., & Fetrow, R. A. (2003). Outcomes during middle school for an elementary school-based preventive intervention for conduct problems: Follow-up results from a randomized trial. *Behavior Therapy, 34,* 525–552.

Elias, M. J. (1995). Primary prevention as health and social competence promotion. *Journal of Primary Prevention, 16,* 5–14.

Ellis, B. J., Boyce, W. T., Belsky, J., Bakermans-Kranenburg, M. J., & van IJzendoorn, M. H. (2011). Differential susceptibility to the environment: An evolutionary, neurodevelopmental theory. *Development and Psychopathology, 23,* 7–28.

Ellis, M. L., Weiss, B., & Lochman, J. E. (2009). Executive functions in children: Associations with aggressive behavior and social appraisal processing. *Journal of Abnormal Child Psychology, 37,* 945–956.

Embretson, S. E., & Reise, S. P. (2000). *Item response theory for psychologists.* Mahwah, NJ: Erlbaum.

Epstein, J. L. (1991). Effects on student achievement of teachers' practices of parent involvement. In S. B. Silvern (Ed.), *Advances in reading/language research: A research annual: Vol. 5. Literacy through family, community, and school interaction* (pp. 261–276). Greenwich, CT: JAI Press.

Estroff, S. E., & Zimmer, C. (1994). Social networks, social support, and violence among persons with severe, persistent mental illness. In J. Monahan & H. Steadman (Eds.), *Violence and mental disorder* (pp. 259–295). Chicago: University of Chicago Press.

Feinberg, M. E., Greenberg, M. T., & Osgood, D. W. (2004). Readiness, functioning, and efficacy in community prevention coalitions: A study of Communities That Care in Pennsylvania. *American Journal of Community Psychology, 33,* 163–176.

Feldman, R. A., Caplinger, T. E., & Wodarski, J. S. (1983). *St. Louis conundrum: The effective treatment of antisocial youths.* Englewood Cliffs, NJ: Prentice Hall.

Fergusson, D. M., Lynskey, M. T., & Horwood, L. J. (1996). Factors associated with continuity and changes in disruptive behavior patterns between childhood and adolescence. *Journal of Abnormal Child Psychology, 24,* 533–553.

Flanagan, C., & Gallay, E. (2014). Adolescents' theories of the "commons." In J. Benson (Ed.), *Advances in child development and behavior* (Vol. 46, pp. 33–55). Oxfordshire, UK: Elsevier.

Flanagan, K. S., Bierman, K. L., Kam, C., & Conduct Problems Prevention Research Group. (2003). Identifying at-risk children at school entry: The usefulness of multi-behavioral problem profiles. *Journal of Clinical Child and Adolescent Psychology, 32,* 396–407.

Flannery-Schroeder, E., & Kendall, P. C. (2000). Group and individual cognitive–behavioral treatments for youth with anxiety disorders: A randomized clinical trial. *Cognitive Therapy and Research, 24,* 251–278.

Forehand, R. L., & McMahon, R. J. (1981). *Helping the noncompliant child: A clinician's guide to parent training.* New York: Guilford Press.

Forehand, R., Middlebrook, J., Rogers, T., & Steffe, M. (1983). Dropping out of parent training. *Behaviour Research and Therapy, 21,* 663–668.

Forman, S. G., Olin, S. S., Hoagwood, K. E., Crowe, M., & Saka, N. (2009). Evidence-based intervention in schools: Developers' views of implementation barriers and facilitators. *School Mental Health: A Multidisciplinary Research and Practice Journal, 1,* 26–36.

Frank, J. L., & Bose, B. K. (2014). Effectiveness of a school-based yoga program on adolescent mental health, stress coping strategies, and attitudes towards violence: Findings from a high-risk sample. *Journal of Applied School Psychology, 30,* 29–49.

Fredrickson, B. L., Grewen, K. M., Algoe, S. B., Firestine, A. M., Arevalo, J. M., Ma, F., & Cole, S. W. (2015). Psychological well-being and the human conserved transcriptional response to adversity. *PLOS ONE, 10,* e0121839.

Frick, P. J., Ray, J. V., Thornton, L. C., & Kahn, R. E. (2014). Can callous-unemotional traits enhance the understanding, diagnosis, and treatment of serious conduct problems in children and adolescents?: A comprehensive review. *Psychological Bulletin, 140,* 1–57.

Glenn, A. L., Lochman, J. E., Dishion, T., Powell, N. P., Boxmeyer, C., Kassing, F., . . . Romero, D. (2019). Toward tailored interventions: Sympathetic and parasympathetic functioning predicts responses to an intervention for conduct problems delivered in two formats. *Prevention Science, 20,* 30–40.

Glenn, A. L., Lochman, J. E., Dishion, T., Powell, N. P., Boxmeyer, C., & Qu, L. (2018). Oxytocin receptor gene variant interacts with intervention delivery format in predicting intervention outcomes for youth with conduct problems. *Prevention Science, 19,* 38–48.

Glueck, S., & Glueck, E. T. (1930). *500 criminal careers.* New York: Knopf.

Goulter, N., Godwin, J., & Conduct Problems Prevention Research Group. (2018, March). *Person-oriented analyses of Fast Track effects: Trajectories for adult criminal convictions.* Poster presented at the Banff International Conference on Behavioural Science, Banff, Alberta, Canada.

Goyal, M., Singh, S., Sibinga, E. M., Gould, N. F., Rowland-Seymour, A., Sharma, R., . . . Haythornthwaite, J. A. (2014). Meditation programs for psychological stress and well-being. *JAMA Internal Medicine, 174,* 357–368.

Granic, I., & Patterson, G. R. (2006). Toward a comprehensive model of antisocial development: A dynamic systems approach. *Psychological Review, 113,* 101–131.

Greenberg, M. T. (2004). Current and future challenges in school-based prevention: The researcher perspective. *Prevention Science, 5,* 5–13.

Greenberg, M. T., & Abenavoli, R. (2017). Universal interventions: Fully exploring their impacts and potential to produce population-level impacts. *Journal of Research on Educational Effectiveness, 1,* 40–67.

Greenberg, M. T., Domitrovich, C. E., Weissberg, R. P., & Durlak, J. A. (2017). Social and emotional learning as a public health approach to education. *The Future of Children, 27,* 13–32.

Greenberg, M. T., & Harris, A. R. (2012). Nurturing mindfulness in children and youth: Current state of research. *Child Development Perspectives, 6,* 161–166.

Greenberg, M. T., Kusché, C. A., & Conduct Problems Prevention Research Group. (2011). *Grade level PATHS (grades 3–4).* South Deerfield, MA: Channing-Bete.

Greenberg, M. T., Kusché, C. A., & Speltz, M. (1991). Emotional regulation, self-control, and psychopathology: The role of relationships in early childhood. In D. Cicchetti & S. L. Toth (Eds.), *Rochester Symposium on Developmental Psychopathology: Vol. 2. Internalizing and externalizing expressions of dysfunction* (pp. 21–66). Hillsdale, NJ: Erlbaum.

Greenberg, M. T., Lengua, L. J., Coie, J. D., Pinderhughes, E. E., & Conduct Problems Prevention Research Group. (1999). Predicting developmental outcomes at school entry using a multiple risk model: Four American communities. *Developmental Psychology, 35,* 403–417.

Greenberg, M. T., & Riggs, N. R. (2015). Prevention of mental disorders and promotion of competence. In A. Tharpar, D. Pine, J. Leckman, M. J. Snowling, S. Scott, & E. Taylor (Eds.), *Rutter's child and adolescent psychiatry* (6th ed., pp. 215–226) West Sussex, UK: Wiley.

Greenberg, M. T., Weissberg, R. P., O'Brien, M. U., Zins, J. E., Fredericks, L., Resnik, H., & Elias, M. J. (2003). Enhancing school-based prevention and youth development through coordinated social, emotional, and academic learning. *American Psychologist, 58,* 466–474.

Grissom, J. A., & Andersen S. (2012). Why superintendents turn over. *American Educational Research Journal, 49,* 1146–1180.

Gross, D., Fogg, L., Webster-Stratton, C., Garvey, C., Julion, W., & Grady, J. (2003). Parent training of toddlers in day care in low-income urban communities. *Journal of Consulting and Clinical Psychology, 71,* 261–278.

Grossman, D. C., Neckerman, H. J., Koepsell, T. D., Liu, P. Y., Asher, K. N., Beland, K., . . . Rivara, F. P. (1997). The effectiveness of a violence prevention curriculum among children in elementary school. *Journal of the American Medical Association, 277,* 1605–1611.

Hahn, R., Fuqua-Whitley, D., Wethington, H., Lowy, J., Crosby, A., Fullilove, M., . . . Price, L. (2007). Effectiveness of universal school-based programs to prevent violent and aggressive behavior: A systematic review. *American Journal of Preventive Medicine, 33*(Suppl. 2), 114–129.

Hall, C. M., & Bierman, K. L. (2015). Technology-assisted interventions for parents of young children: Emerging practices, current research, and future directions. *Early Childhood Research Quarterly, 33,* 21–32.

Hansen, W. B., Graham, J. W., Wolkenstein, B., & Lundy, B. Z. (1988). Differential impact of three alcohol prevention curricula on hypothesized mediating variables. *Journal of Drug Education, 18,* 143–153.

Hawkins, J. D., Catalano, R. F., Kosterman, R., Abbott, R., & Hill, K. G. (1999). Preventing adolescent health-risk behaviors by strengthening protection during childhood. *Archives of Pediatric Adolescent Medicine, 153,* 226–234.

Hawkins, J. D., Kosterman, R., Catalano, R. F., Hill, K. G., & Abbott, R. D. (2005). Promoting positive adult functioning through social development intervention in childhood. *Archives of Pediatrics and Adolescent Medicine, 159,* 25–31.

Hawkins, J. D., & Weiss, J. G. (1985). The Social Development Model: An integrated approach to delinquency prevention. *Journal of Primary Prevention, 6,* 73–95.

Healy, W., & Bronner, A. F. (1948). What makes a child delinquent? In N. B. Henry (Ed.), *Forty-seventh yearbook of the National Society for Study of Education* (pp. 30–47). Chicago: University of Chicago Press.

Heckman, J. J., Pinto, F., & Savelyev, P. (2013). Understanding the mechanisms through which an influential early childhood program boosted adult outcomes. *American Economic Review, 103,* 2052–2086.

Henderson, A. T., & Mapp, K. L. (2002). *A new wave of evidence: The impact of school, family and community connections on student achievement* (Research Synthesis). Austin, TX: National Center for Family and Community Connections with Schools.

Henggeler, S. W. (2011). Efficiency studies to large-scale transport: The development and variation of Multisystemic Therapy programs. *Annual Review of Clinical Psychology, 7,* 351–381.

Henggeler, S. W., Schoenwald, S. K., & Pickrel, S. G. (1995). Multisystemic Therapy: Bridging the gap between university- and community-based treatment. *Journal of Consulting and Clinical Psychology, 63,* 709–717.

Henry, D., Guerra, N., Huesmann, R., Tolan, P., VanAcker, R., & Eron, L. (2000). Normative influences on aggression in urban elementary school classrooms. *American Journal of Community Psychology, 28,* 59–81.

Herrnstein, R. J., & Murray, C. (1994). *The bell curve: Intelligence and class structure in American life.* New York: Simon & Schuster.

Hill, L. G., Lochman, J. E., & Conduct Problems Prevention Research Group. (2004). Effectiveness of kindergarten and first-grade screening for conduct problems in sixth grade. *Journal of Consulting and Clinical Psychology, 72,* 809–820.

Hinshaw, S. P. (1992). Externalizing behavior problems and academic underachievement in childhood and adolescence: Causal relationships and underlying mechanisms. *Psychological Bulletin, 111,* 127–155.

Holbein, J. B. (2017). Childhood skill development and adult political participation. *American Political Science Review, 111,* 572–583.

Hollingshead, A. B. (1975). *Four factor index of social status.* New Haven, CT: Yale University.

Hölzel, B. K., Lazar, S. W., Gard, T., Schuman-Olivier, Z., Vago, D. R., & Ott, U. (2011). How does mindfulness meditation work? Proposing mechanisms of action from a conceptual and neural perspective. *Perspectives on Psychological Science, 6,* 537–559.

Hubbard, J. A., Smithmyer, C. M., Ramsden, S. R., Parker, E. H., Flanagan, K. D., Dearing, K. F., . . . Simons, R. F. (2002). Observational, physiological, and self-report measures of children's anger: Relations to reactive versus proactive aggression. *Child Development, 73,* 1101–1118.

Hughes, J. N., Cavell, T. A., Meehan, B. T., Zhang, D., & Collie, C. (2005). Adverse school context moderates the outcomes of selective interventions for aggressive children. *Journal of Consulting and Clinical Psychology, 73,* 731–736.

Humphreys, L., Forehand, R., McMahon, R. J., & Roberts, M. (1978). Parent behavioral training to modify child noncompliance: Effects on untreated siblings. *Journal of Behavior Therapy and Experimental Psychiatry, 9,* 235–238.

Jennings, W. G., Rocque, M., Fox, B. H., Piquero, A. R., & Farrington, D. P. (2016). Can they recover?: An assessment of adult adjustment problems among males in the abstainer, recovery, life-course-persistent and adolescence-limited pathways followed up to age 56 in the Cambridge Study in Delinquent Development. *Development and Psychopathology, 28,* 537–549.

Jimerson, S. R., & Ferguson, P. (2007). A longitudinal study of grade retention: Academic and behavioral outcomes of retained students through adolescence. *School Psychology Quarterly, 22,* 314–339.

Jones, D., Dodge, K. A., Foster, E. M., Nix, R., & Conduct Problems Prevention Research Group. (2002). Early identification of children at risk for costly mental health service use. *Prevention Science, 3,* 247–256.

Jones, D., Godwin, J., Dodge, K. A., Bierman, K. L., Coie, J. D., Greenberg, M. T., . . . Pinderhughes, E. E. (2010). Impact of the Fast Track prevention program on health services use by conduct-problem youth. *Pediatrics, 125,* e130–e136.

Jones, D. E., Greenberg, M., & Crowley, M. (2015). Early social-emotional functioning and public health: The relationship between kindergarten social competence and future wellness. *American Journal of Public Health, 105,* 2283–2290.

Jones, D. J., Forehand, R. L., Cuellar, J., Parent, J., & Honeycutt, A. A. (2014). Technology-enhanced program for child disruptive behavior disorders: Development and pilot randomized control trial. *Journal of Clinical Child and Adolescent Psychology, 43,* 88–101.

Kabat-Zinn, J. (1990). *Full catastrophe living: Using the wisdom of your body and mind to face stress, pain, and illness.* New York: Dell.

Karver, M. S., Handelsman, J. B., Fields, S., & Bickman, L. (2005). A theoretical model of common process factors in youth and family therapy. *Mental Health Services Research, 7,* 35–51.

Kassing, F., Godwin, J., Lochman, J. E., Coie, J. D., & Conduct Problems Prevention Research Group. (2019). Using early childhood behavior problems to predict adult convictions. *Journal of Abnormal Child Psychology, 47,* 765–778.

Kazdin, A. E. (1987). Treatment of antisocial behavior in children: Current status and future directions. *Psychological Bulletin, 102,* 187–203.

Kazdin, A. E. (1993). Treatment of conduct disorder: Progress and directions in psychotherapy research. *Development and Psychopathology, 5,* 277–310.

Keenan, K., Loeber, R., Zhang, Q., Stouthamer-Loeber, M., & Van Kammen, W. B. (1995). The influence of deviant peers on the development of boys' disruptive and delinquent behavior: A temporal analysis. *Development and Psychopathology, 7,* 715–726.

Kendziora, K., & Osher, D. (2016). Promoting children's and adolescents' social and emotional development: District adaptations of a theory of action. *Journal of Clinical Child and Adolescent Psychology, 45,* 797–811.

Kerr, M., & Stattin, H. (2000). What parents know, how they know it, and several forms of adolescent adjustment: Further support for a reinterpretation of monitoring. *Developmental Psychology, 36,* 366–380.

Kim, B. K. E., Gloppen, K. M., Rhew, I. C., Oesterle, S., & Hawkins, J. D. (2015). Effects of the Communities That Care prevention system on youth reports of protective factors. *Prevention Science, 16,* 652–662.

Kimonis, E., Frick, P. J., & McMahon, R. J. (2014). Conduct and oppositional defiant disorders. In E. J. Mash & R. A. Barkley (Eds.), *Child psychopathology* (3rd ed., pp. 145–179). New York: Guilford Press.

Klingbeil, D. A., Renshaw, T. L., Willenbrink, J. B., Copek, R. A., Chan, K. T., Haddock, A., . . . Clifton, J. (2017). Mindfulness-based interventions with youth: A comprehensive meta-analysis of group-design studies. *Journal of School Psychology, 63,* 77–103.

Kratochwill, T. R., Volpiansky, P., Clements, M., & Ball, C. (2007). Professional development in implementing and sustaining multitier prevention models: Implications for response to intervention. *School Psychology Review, 36,* 618–631.

Krisberg, B. (2005). *Juvenile justice: Redeeming our children.* Thousand Oaks, CA: SAGE.

Kusché, C. A., Greenberg, M. T., & Conduct Problems Prevention Research Group. (2011). *Grade level PATHS (grades 1–2).* South Deerfield, MA: Channing-Bete.

Lahey, B. B., Loeber, R., Burke, J., & Rathouz, P. J. (2002). Adolescent outcomes of childhood conduct disorder among clinic-referred boys: Predictors of improvement. *Journal of Abnormal Child Psychology, 30,* 333–348.

Landau, S., Milich, R., & Diener, M. B. (1998). Peer relations of children with attention-deficit hyperactivity disorder. *Reading and Writing Quarterly: Overcoming Learning Difficulties, 14,* 83–105.

Lavallee, K. L., Bierman, K. L., Nix, R. L., & Conduct Problems Prevention Research Group. (2005). The impact of first-grade "Friendship Group" experiences on child social outcomes in the Fast Track program. *Journal of Abnormal Child Psychology, 33,* 307–324.

Lightfoot, M., Rotheram-Borus, M., Comulada, W. S., Reddy, V. S., & Duan, N. (2010). Efficacy of brief interventions in clinical care settings for persons living with HIV. *Journal of Acquired Immune Deficiency Syndromes, 53,* 348–356.

Lipsey, M. W. (2006). The effects of community-based group treatment for delinquency: A meta-analytic search for cross-study generalizations. In K.

A. Dodge, T. J. Dishion, & J. E. Lansford (Eds.), *Deviant peer influences in programs for youth: Problems and solutions* (pp. 162–184). New York: Guilford Press.

Lochman, J. E., Boxmeyer, C. L., Jones, S., Qu, L., Ewoldsen, D., & Nelson, W. M., III. (2017). Testing the feasibility of a briefer school-based preventive intervention with aggressive children: A hybrid intervention with face-to-face and internet components. *Journal of School Psychology, 62,* 33–50.

Lochman, J. E., Coie, J. D., Underwood, M. K., & Terry, R. (1993). Effectiveness of a social relations intervention program for aggressive and nonaggressive, rejected children. *Journal of Consulting and Clinical Psychology, 61,* 1053–1058.

Lochman, J. E., & Conduct Problems Prevention Research Group. (1995). Screening of child behavior problems for prevention programs at school entry. *Journal of Consulting and Clinical Psychology, 63,* 549–559.

Lochman, J. E., Dishion, T. J., Boxmeyer, C. L., Powell, N. P., & Qu, L. (2017). Variations in response to evidence-based group preventive intervention for disruptive behavior problems: A view from 938 Coping Power sessions. *Journal of Abnormal Child Psychology, 45,* 1271–1284.

Lochman, J. E., Dishion, T. J., Powell, N. P., Boxmeyer, C. L., Qu, L., & Sallee, M. (2015). Evidence-based preventive intervention for preadolescent aggressive children: One-year outcomes following randomization to group versus individual delivery. *Journal of Consulting and Clinical Psychology, 83,* 728–735.

Lochman, J. E., Powell, N. R., Jackson, M. F., & Czopp, W. (2006). Cognitive-behavioral psychotherapy for conduct disorder: The Coping Power program. In W. M. Nelson, III, A. J. Finch, Jr., & K. J. Hart (Eds.), *Conduct disorders: A practitioner's guide to comparative treatments* (pp. 177–215). New York: Springer.

Lochman, J. E., & Wells, K. C. (2002). Contextual social-cognitive mediators and child outcome: A test of the theoretical model in the coping power program. *Development and Psychopathology, 14,* 945–967.

Lochman, J. E., & Wells, K. C. (2004). The Coping Power program for preadolescent aggressive boys and their parents: Outcome effects at the one-year follow-up. *Journal of Consulting and Clinical Psychology, 72,* 571–578.

Lochman, J. E., Wells, K. C., Qu, L., & Chen, L. (2013). Three year follow-up of coping power intervention effects: Evidence of neighborhood moderation? *Prevention Science, 14,* 364–376.

Loeber, R., & Dishion, T. J. (1983). Early predictors of male delinquency: A review. *Psychological Bulletin, 74,* 68–99.

Loeber, R., Lahey, B. B., & Thomas, C. (1991). Diagnostic conundrum of oppositional defiant disorder and conduct disorder. *Journal of Abnormal Psychology, 100,* 379–390.

Lopez-Duran, N., Olson, S. L., Hajal, N. J., Felt, B. T., & Vazquez, D. M. (2009). Hypothalamic pituitary adrenal axis functioning in reactive and proactive aggression in children. *Journal of Abnormal Child Psychology, 37,* 169–182.

Lösel, F., & Beelmann, A. (2003). Effects of child skills training in preventing antisocial behavior: A systematic review of randomized evaluations. *Annals of the AAPSS, 587,* 84–109.

Lundahl, B. W., Risser, H. J., & Lovejoy, M. C. (2006). A meta-analysis of parent training: Moderators and follow-up effects. *Clinical Psychology Review, 26,* 86–104.

Luthar, S. S., & Zigler, E. (1991). Vulnerability and competence: A review of research on resilience in childhood. *American Journal of Orthopsychiatry, 61,* 6–22.

Lytton, H. (1990). Child and parent effects in boys' conduct disorder: A re-interpretation. *Developmental Psychology, 26,* 683–697.

MacDonell, K. W., & Prinz, R. J. (2017). A review of technology-based youth and family-focused interventions. *Clinical Child and Family Psychology Review, 20,* 185–200.

Mager, W., Milich, R., Harris, M. J., & Howard, A. (2005). Intervention groups for adolescents with conduct problems: Is aggregation harmful or helpful? *Journal of Abnormal Child Psychology, 33,* 349–362.

Maggs, J. L., & Schulenberg, J. (2001). Editors' introduction: Prevention as altering the course of development and the complementary purposes of developmental and prevention sciences. *Applied Developmental Science, 5,* 196–200.

Manassis, K., Mendlowitz, S. L., Scapillato, D., Avery, D., Fiksenbaum, L., Freire, M., . . . Owens, M. (2002). Group and individual cognitive-behavioral therapy for childhood anxiety disorders: A randomized trial. *Journal of the American Academy of Child and Adolescent Psychiatry, 41,* 1423–1430.

Markus, H., & Nurius, P. (1986). Possible selves. *American Psychologist, 41,* 954–969.

Marwick, C. (1992). Guns, drugs threaten to raise public health problem of violence to epidemic. *Journal of the American Medical Association, 267,* 2993.

Matthys, W., Vanderschuren, L. J. M. J., Schutter, D. J. L. G., & Lochman, J. E. (2012). Impaired neurocognitive functions affect social learning processes in oppositional defiant disorder and conduct disorder: Implications for interventions. *Clinical Child and Family Psychology Review, 15,* 234–246.

Maynard, B. R., Solis, M., Miller, V., & Brendel, K. E. (2017). Mindfulness-based interventions for improving academic achievement, behavior and socio-emotional functioning of primary and secondary students: A systematic review. Retrieved from *www.campbellcollaboration.org/library/mindfulness-based-interventions-primary-and-secondary-school-students.html.*

McCord, J. (1978). A thirty-year follow-up of treatment effects. *American Psychologist, 2,* 284–289.

McCord, J. (1992). The Cambridge–Sommerville Study: A pioneering longitudinal-experimental study of delinquency prevention. In J. McCord & R. Tremblay (Eds.), *Preventing antisocial behavior: Interventions from birth to adolescence* (pp. 196–209). New York: Guilford Press.

McCord, J., Tremblay, R. E., Vitaro, F., & Desmarais-Gervais, L. (1994). Boys' disruptive behaviour, school adjustment, and delinquency: The Montreal Prevention Experiment. *International Journal of Behavioral Development, 17,* 739–752.

McFall, R. M., & Treat, T. A. (1999). Quantifying the information value of clinical assessments with signal detection theory. *Annual Review of Psychology, 50,* 215–241.

McGoron, L., & Ondersma, S. J. (2015). Reviewing the need for technological and other expansions of evidence-based parent training for young children. *Child and Youth Services Review, 59,* 71–83.

McGowan, H. M., Nix, R. L., Murphy, S. A., Bierman, K. L., & Conduct Problems Prevention Research Group. (2010). Investigating the impact of selection bias in dose-response analyses of preventive interventions. *Prevention Science, 11,* 239–251.

McMahon, R. J., & Forehand, R. L. (2003). *Helping the noncompliant child: Family-based treatment for oppositional behavior* (2nd ed.). New York: Guilford Press.

McMahon, R. J., & Frick, P. J. (2019). Conduct and oppositional disorders. In M. J. Prinstein, E. A. Youngstrom, E. J. Mash, & R. A. Barkley (Eds.), *Treatment of childhood disorders* (4th ed., pp. 102–172). New York: Guilford Press.

McMahon, R. J., Katz, L. F., Kerns, S. E. U., Pasalich, D. S., Pullmann, M. D., Gurtovenko, K., . . . Dorsey, S. (2018, July). Parent management training and emotion coaching for children with callous-unemotional traits: A treatment development study. In R. J. McMahon (Chair), *New directions in the assessment and treatment of children with conduct problems and callous-unemotional traits.* Symposium presented at the meeting of the International Society for the Study of Behavioural Development, Gold Coast, Australia.

McMahon, R. J., Slough, N., & Conduct Problems Prevention Research Group. (1996). Family-based intervention in the Fast Track program. In R. D. Peters & R. J. McMahon (Eds.), *Preventing childhood disorders, substance use, and delinquency* (pp. 90–110). Newbury Park, CA: SAGE.

McMahon, R. J., Slough, N., Lochman, J. E., Dodge, K. A., Coie, J. D., Bierman, K. L., & Greenberg, M. T. (2019). *The Fast Track Parent Group manual.* Manuscript submitted for publication.

McMahon, R. J., Wells, K. C., & Kotler, J. S. (2006). In E. J. Mash & R. A. Barkley (Eds.), *Treatment of childhood disorders* (3rd ed., pp. 137–268). New York: Guilford Press.

McMahon, R. J., Witkiewitz, K., Kotler, J. S., & Conduct Problems Prevention Research Group. (2010). Predictive validity of callous-unemotional traits measured in early adolescence with respect to multiple antisocial outcomes. *Journal of Abnormal Psychology, 119,* 752–763.

McMahon, R. J., Witkiewitz, J., & Wu, J. (2009). *Fast Track intervention reduced the substance use of white youth, who smoked fewer cigarettes, drank less alcohol, did less binge drinking and used less marijuana than youth in the control group.* Unpublished report.

Meany, M. J. (2001). Maternal care, gene expression, and the transmission of individual differences in stress reactivity across generations. *Annual Review of Neuroscience, 24,* 1161–1192.

Mendelson, T., Dariotis, J. K., Feagans Gould, L., Smith, A. S., Smith, A. A. Gonzalez, A. A., & Greenberg, M. T. (2013). Implementing mindfulness and yoga in urban schools: A community–academic partnership. *Journal of Children's Services, 8,* 276–291.

Miller, S., Boxmeyer, C. L., Lochman, J. E., Romero, D., Powell, N., & Jones, S. (2018, June). Optimizing the Coping Power preventive intervention for children with reactive aggression by integrating mindfulness. In S. Miller (Chair), *Effectiveness studies of mindfulness with children, parents, and teachers.* Symposium conducted at the meeting of the Society for Prevention Research, Washington, DC.

Mind and Life Education Research Network. (2012). Contemplative practices and mental training: Prospects for American education. *Child Development Perspectives, 6,* 146–153.

Moffitt, T. E. (1993). Adolescence-limited and life-course-persistent antisocial behavior: A development taxonomy. *Psychological Review, 100,* 674–701.

Molina, B. S. G., Flory, K., Bukstein, O. G., Greiner, A. R., Baker, J. L., Krug, V., & Evans, S. W. (2008). Feasibility and preliminary efficacy of an after-school program for middle schoolers with ADHD: A randomized trial in a large public middle school. *Journal of Attention Disorders, 12,* 207–217.

Molina, B. S. G., Hinshaw, S. P., Swanson, J. M., Arnold, L. E., Vitiello, B., Jensen, P. S., . . . Houck, P. R. (2009). The MTA at 8 years: Prospective follow-up of children treated for combined-type ADHD in a multisite study. *Journal of the American Academy of Child and Adolescent Psychiatry, 48,* 484–500.

Mrazek, P. J., Haggerty, R. J., & National Academy of Sciences Institute of Medicine, Division of Biobehavioral Sciences & Mental Disorders, Committee on Prevention of Mental Disorders. (1994). *Reducing risks for mental disorders: Frontiers for preventive intervention research.* Washington, DC: National Academy Press.

National Center for Injury Prevention and Control. (1992). The prevention of youth violence: A framework for community action. Retrieved September 11, 2018, from *https://wonder.cdc.gov/wonder/prevguid/p0000026/p0000026.asp.*

Nix, R. L., Bierman, K. L., McMahon, R. J., & Conduct Problems Prevention Research Group. (2009). How attendance and quality of participation affect treatment response in parent behavior management training. *Journal of Consulting and Clinical Psychology, 77,* 429–438.

Nix, R. L., Pinderhughes, E. E., Bierman, K. L., Maples, J. J., & Conduct Problems Prevention Research Group. (2005). Decoupling the relation between risk factors for conduct problems and the receipt of intervention services: Participation across multiple components of a prevention program. *American Journal of Community Psychology, 36,* 307–325.

Odgers, C. L., Caspi, A., Broadbent, J. M., Dickson, N., Hancox, R. J., Harrington, H., . . . Moffitt, T. E. (2007). Prediction of differential adult health burden by conduct problem subtypes in males. *Archives of General Psychiatry, 64*, 476–484.

O'Donnell, J., Hawkins, J. D., Catalano, R. F., Abbott, R. D., & Day, L. E. (1995). Preventing school failure, drug use, and delinquency among low-income children: Long-term intervention in elementary schools. *American Journal of Orthopsychiatry, 65*, 87–100.

Offord, D. R. (2000). Selection levels of prevention. *Addictive Behaviors, 25*, 833–842.

Offord, D. R., Boyle, M. C., & Racine, Y. A. (1991). The epidemiology of anti-social behavior in childhood and adolescence. In D. J. Pepler & K. H. Rubin (Eds.), *The development and treatment of childhood aggression* (pp. 31–54). Hillsdale, NJ: Erlbaum.

OJJDP Statistical Briefing Book. (n.d.). Retrieved October 22, 2018, from *www. ojjdp.gov/ojstatbb/crime/JAR_Display.asp?ID=qa05200*.

Olds, D., Henderson, C. R., Cole, R., Eckenrode, J., Kitzman, H., Luckey, D., . . . Powers, J. (1998). Long-term effects of nurse home visitation on chil-dren's criminal and antisocial behavior. *Journal of the American Medical Association, 280*, 1238–1244.

Orrell-Valente, J. K., Pinderhughes, E. E., Valente, E., Laird, R. D., & Con-duct Problems Prevention Research Group. (1999). If it's offered, will they come?: Influences on parents' participation in a community-based conduct problems prevention program. *American Journal of Community Psychol-ogy, 27*, 753–783.

Oyserman, D., & Markus, H. (1993). The socio-cultural self. In J. Suls (Ed.), *Psychological perspective on the self* (Vol. 14, pp. 187–220). Hillsdale, NJ: Erlbaum.

Oyserman, D., Terry, K., & Bybee, D. (2002). A possible selves intervention to enhance school involvement. *Journal of Adolescence, 25*, 313–326.

Pardini, D. A., Lochman, J. E., & Powell, N. (2007). Shared or unique devel-opmental pathways to callous-unemotional traits and antisocial behavior in children? *Journal of Clinical Child and Adolescent Psychology, 36*, 319–333.

Pasalich, D. S., Witkiewitz, K., McMahon, R. J., Pinderhughes, E. E., & Con-duct Problems Prevention Research Group. (2016). Indirect effects of the Fast Track intervention on conduct disorder symptoms and callous-unemotional traits: Distinct pathways involving discipline and warmth. *Journal of Abnormal Child Psychology, 44*, 587–597.

Patterson, G. R., Reid, J. B., & Dishion, T. J. (1992). *Antisocial boys*. Eugene, OR: Castalia.

Paunesku, D., Walton, G. M., Romero, C., Smith, E. N., Yeager, D. S., & Dweck, C. S. (2015). Mind-set interventions are a scalable treatment for academic underachievement. *Psychological Science, 26*, 784–793.

Pentz, M. A., Trebow, E. A., Hansen, W. B., MacKinnon, D. P., Dwyer, J. H., Johnson, C., . . . Cormack, C. (1990). Effects of program implementa-tion on adolescent drug use behavior: The Midwestern Prevention Project. *Evaluation Review, 14*, 264–289.

Perroud, N., Baud, P., Ardu, S., Krejci, I., Mouthon, D., Vessaz, M., . . . Courtet, P. (2013). Temperament personality profiles in suicidal behaviour: An investigation of associated demographic, clinical and genetic factors. *Journal of Affective Disorders, 146,* 246–253.

Pfiffner, L., Rooney, M., Haack, L., Villodas, M., Delucchi, K., & McBurnett, K. (2016). A randomized controlled trial of a school-implemented school–home intervention for attention-deficit/hyperactivity disorder symptoms and impairment. *Journal of the American Academy of Child and Adolescent Psychiatry, 55,* 762–770.

Piotrowska, P. J., Tully, L. A., Lenroot, R., Kimonis, E., Hawes, D., Moul, C., . . . Dadds, M. R. (2017). Mothers, fathers, and parental systems: A conceptual model of parental engagement in programmes for child mental health—Connect, Attend, Participate, Enact (CAPE). *Clinical Child and Family Psychology Review, 20,* 146–161.

Pollard, J. A., Hawkins, J. D., & Arthur, M. W. (1999). Risk and protection: Are both necessary to understand diverse behavioral outcomes in adolescence? *Social Work Research, 23,* 145–158.

Poulin, F., Dishion, T. J., & Burraston, B. (2001). 3-year iatrogenic effects associated with aggregating high-risk adolescents in cognitive-behavioral preventive interventions. *Applied Developmental Science, 5,* 214–224.

Powers, C. J., Bierman, K. L., & Coffman, D. (2016). Restrictive educational placements for students with early-starting conduct problems: Associations with high-school non-completion and adolescent maladjustment. *Journal of Child Psychology and Psychiatry, 57,* 899–908.

Protzko, J. (2015). The environment in raising early intelligence: A meta-analysis of the fadeout effect. *Intelligence, 53,* 202–210.

Public Health Service. (1990). *Healthy people 2000: National health promotion and disease prevention objectives.* Washington, DC: U.S. Department of Health and Human Services, Public Health Service.

Rabiner, D. L., Malone, P. S., & Conduct Problems Prevention Research Group. (2004). The impact of tutoring on early reading achievement for children with and without attention problems. *Journal of Abnormal Child Psychology, 32,* 273–284.

Racz, S. J., King, K. M., Wu, J., Witkiewitz, K., McMahon, R. J., & Conduct Problems Prevention Research Group. (2013). The predictive utility of a brief kindergarten screening measure of child behavior problems. *Journal of Consulting and Clinical Psychology, 81,* 588–599.

Racz, S. J., & McMahon, R. J. (2011). The relationship between parental knowledge and monitoring and child and adolescent conduct problems: A 10-year update. *Clinical Child and Family Psychology Review, 14,* 377–398.

Racz, S., McMahon, R. J., & Luthar, S. S. (2011). Risky behavior in affluent youth: Examining the co-occurrence and consequences of multiple problem behaviors. *Journal of Child and Family Studies, 20,* 120–128.

Robbins, M. S., Turner, C. W., Alexander, J. F., & Perez, G. A. (2003). Alliance and dropout in family therapy for adolescents with behavior problems: Individual and systemic effects. *Journal of Family Psychology, 17,* 534–544.

Roberts, S., Lester, K. J., Hudson, J. L., Rapee, R. M., Creswell, C., Cooper, P. J., . . . Eley, T. C. (2014). Serotonin transporter methylation and response to cognitive behavior therapy in children with anxiety disorders. *Translational Psychiatry, 4*, e444.

Robins, L. (1978). Sturdy childhood predictors of adult antisocial behavior: Replications from longitudinal studies. *Psychological Medicine, 8*, 611–622.

Sampson, R. J. (2017). Breaking the cycle of compounded adversity in the lives of institutionalized youth. *JAMA Pediatrics, 171*, 111–113.

Sanders, M. R. (2012). Development, evaluation, and multinational dissemination of the Triple P-Positive Parenting Program. *Annual Review of Clinical Psychology, 8*, 345–379.

Sanders, M. R., Baker, S., & Turner, K. M. T. (2012). A randomized controlled trial evaluating the efficacy of Triple P Online with parents of children with early-onset conduct problems. *Behaviour Research and Therapy, 50*, 675–684.

Sanders, M. R., & Markie-Dadds, C. (1992). Toward a technology of prevention of disruptive behaviour disorders: The role of behavioural family intervention. *Behaviour Change, 9*, 186–200.

Schechtman, Z., & Ben-David, M. (1999). Individual and group psychotherapy of childhood aggression: A comparison of outcomes and process. *Group Dynamics: Theory, Research, and Practice, 3*, 263–274.

Scheffler, R. M., Brown, T. T., Fulton, B. D., Hinshaw, S. P., Levine, P., & Stone, S. (2009). Positive association between attention-deficit/hyperactivity disorder medication use and academic achievement during elementary school. *Pediatrics, 123*, 1273–1279.

Schofield, H. T. (2009). *Predicting change in conduct problems during middle school: The utility of risk and protective factors assessed during middle school.* Unpublished dissertation, Pennsylvania State University.

Schofield, H. T., Bierman, K. L., Heinrichs, B., Nix, R. L., & Conduct Problems Prevention Research Group. (2008). Predicting early sexual activity with behavior problems exhibited at school entry and in early adolescence. *Journal of Abnormal Child Psychology, 36*, 1175–1188.

Shaffer, D., Fisher, P., Lucas, C., & Comer, J. (2003). *Scoring manual: Diagnostic Interview Schedule for Children (DISC-IV).* New York: Columbia University.

Sherman, L. J. (2007). The power few: Experimental criminology and the reduction of harm. *Journal of Experimental Criminology, 3*, 299–321.

Singh, N. N., Lancioni, G. E., Joy, S. D. S., Winton, A. S. W., Sabaawi, M., Wahler, R. G., & Singh, J. (2007). Adolescents with conduct disorder can be mindful of their aggressive behavior. *Journal of Emotional and Behavioral Disorders, 15*, 56–63.

Sorensen, L. C., Dodge, K. A., & Conduct Problems Prevention Research Group. (2015). How does the Fast Track intervention prevent adverse outcomes in young adulthood? *Child Development, 87*, 429–445.

Stattin, H., & Kerr, M. (2000). Parental monitoring: A reinterpretation. *Child Development, 71*, 1072–1085.

Steele, C. M., & Aronson, J. (1995). Stereotype threat and the intellectual test-performance of African-Americans. *Journal of Personality and Social Psychology, 69,* 797–811.

Stephan, S. H., Sugai, G., Lever, N., & Connors, E. (2015). Strategies for integrating mental health into schools via a multi-tiered system of support. *School Mental Health, 24,* 211–232.

Stouthamer-Loeber, M., Loeber, R., Wei, E. Farrington, D. P., & Wikstrom, P. H. (2002). Risk and promotive effects in the explanation of persistent serious delinquency in boys. *Journal of Consulting and Clinical Psychology, 70,* 111–123.

Tang, Y., Ma, Y., Wang, J., Fan, Y., Feng, S., Lu, Q., . . . Posner, M. I. (2007). Short-term meditation training improves attention and self-regulation. *PNAS Proceedings of the National Academy of Sciences of the United States of America, 104,* 17152–17156.

Taylor, T. K., Webster-Stratton, C., Feil, E. G., Broadbent, B., Widdop, C. S., & Severson, H. H. (2008). Computer-based intervention with coaching: An example using the Incredible Years program. *Cognitive Behaviour Therapy, 37,* 233–246.

Thornberry, T. P. (1987). Toward an interactional theory of delinquency. *Criminology, 25,* 863–891.

Thornberry, T. P., Huizinga, D., & Loeber, R. (1995). The prevention of serious delinquency and violence: Implications from the program of research on the causes and correlates of delinquency. In J. C. Howell, B. Krisberg, J. D. Hawkins, & J. J. Wilson (Eds.), *A sourcebook: Serious, violent, and chronic juvenile offenders* (pp. 213–237). Thousand Oaks, CA: SAGE.

Tracy, P. E., Wolfgang, M. E., & Figlio, R. M. (1990). *Delinquency careers in two birth cohorts.* New York: Springer.

Tremblay, R. E., Pagani-Kurtz, L., Masse, L. C., Vitaro, F., & Pihl, R. O. (1995). A bi-modal preventive intervention for disruptive kindergarten boys: Its impact through mid-adolescence. *Journal of Consulting and Clinical Psychology, 63,* 560–568.

U.S. Department of Education, National Center for Education Statistics. (2001). Public Elementary/Secondary School Universe Survey, 1999–2000, and Local Education Agency Universe Survey, 1999–2000. Retrieved from *http://nces.ed.gov/pubs2001/100_largest/discussion.asp#tableC.*

Vitaro, F., Brendgen, M., Giguère, C., & Tremblay, R. E. (2013). Early prevention of life-course personal and property violence: A 19-year follow-up of the Montreal Longitudinal–Experimental Study (MLES). *Journal of Experimental Criminology, 9,* 411–427.

Walker, H., Colvin, G., & Ramsey, E. (1996). Antisocial behavior in school: Strategies and best practices. *Behavior Disorders, 21,* 248–256.

Walker, H., Stiller, B., Severson, H. H., Feil, E. G., & Golly, A. (1998). First Step to Success: Intervening at the point of school entry to prevent antisocial behavior patterns. *Psychology in the Schools, 35,* 259–269.

Wallach, M. A., & Wallach, L. (1976). *Teaching all children to read.* Chicago: University of Chicago Press.

Wasik, B. A., & Slavin, R. E. (1993). Preventing early reading failure with one-to-one tutoring: A review of five programs. *Reading Research Quarterly, 28,* 179–200.

Wasik, B. H., Bryant, D. M., & Lyons, C. M. (1990). *Home visiting: Procedures for helping families.* Newbury Park, CA: SAGE.

Webster-Stratton, C. (1984). Randomized trial of two parent-training programs for families with conduct-disordered children. *Journal of Consulting and Clinical Psychology, 52,* 666–678.

Weiss, B., Caron, A., Ball, S., Tapp, J., Johnson, M., & Weisz, J. R. (2005). Iatrogenic effects of group treatment for antisocial youths. *Journal of Consulting and Clinical Psychology, 73,* 1036–1044.

Weissberg, R. P., & Greenberg, M. T. (1998). School and community competence-enhancement and prevention programs. In W. Damon (Series Ed.), I. E. Sigel & K. A. Renninger (Vol. Eds.), *Handbook of child psychology: Vol 4. Child psychology in practice* (5th ed., pp. 877–954). New York: Wiley.

Werthamer-Larsson, L., Kellam, S. G., & Wheeler, L. (1991). Effect of first-grade classroom environment on shy behavior, aggressive behavior, and concentration problems. *American Journal of Community Psychology, 19,* 585–602.

West, D. J., & Farrington, D. P. (1973). *Who becomes delinquent?* London: Heinemann Educational.

Westen, D., & Weinberger, J. (2004). When clinical description becomes statistical prediction. *American Psychologist, 59,* 595–613.

Williams, S. C., Lochman, J. E., Phillips, N. C., & Barry, T. D. (2003). Aggressive and nonaggressive boys' physiological and cognitive processes in response to peer provocations. *Journal of Clinical Child and Adolescent Psychology, 32,* 568–576.

Wilson, S. J., & Lipsey, M. W. (2007). School-based interventions for aggressive and disruptive behavior: Update of a meta-analysis. *American Journal of Preventative Medicine, 33,* S130–S143.

Wright, J. C., Giammarino, M., & Parad, H. W. (1986). Social status in small groups: Individual group similarity and the social "misfit." *Journal of Personality and Social Psychology, 50,* 523–536.

Wu, J., King, K. M., Witkiewitz, K., Racz, S. J., McMahon, R. J., & Conduct Problems Prevention Research Group. (2012). Item analysis and differential item functioning of a brief conduct problem screen. *Psychological Assessment, 24,* 444–454.

Wu, J., Witkiewitz, K., McMahon, R. J., Dodge, K. A., & Conduct Problems Prevention Research Group. (2010). A parallel process growth mixture model of conduct problems and substance use with risky sexual behavior. *Drug and Alcohol Dependence, 111,* 207–214.

Yeager, D. S., Johnson, R., Spitzer, B. J., Trzesniewski, K. H., Powers, J., & Dweck, C. S. (2014). The far-reaching effects of believing people can change: Implicit theories of personality shape stress, health, and achievement during adolescence. *Journal of Personality and Social Psychology, 106,* 867–884.

Yehuda, R., Daskalakis, N. P., Desarnaud, F., Makotkine, I., Lehrner, A. L.,

Koch, E., . . . Bierer, L. M. (2013). Epigenetic biomarkers as predictors and correlates of symptom improvement following psychotherapy in combat veterans with PTSD. *Frontiers in Psychiatry, 4.*

Zheng, Y., Albert, D., McMahon, R. J., Dodge, K., Dick, D., & Conduct Problems Prevention Research Group. (2018). Glucocorticoid receptor (*NR3C1*) gene polymorphism moderate intervention effects on the developmental trajectory of African-American adolescent alcohol abuse. *Prevention Science, 19,* 79–89.

Zimmer-Gembeck, M., & Collins, W. A. (2003). Autonomy development during adolescence. In G. R. Adams & M. D. Berzonsky (Eds.), *Blackwell handbook of adolescence* (pp. 175–204). Malden, MA: Blackwell.

Zoccolillo, M., Tremblay, R., & Vitaro, F. (1996). DSM-III-R and DSM-III criteria for conduct disorder in preadolescent girls: Specific but insensitive. *Journal of the American Academy of Child and Adolescent Psychiatry, 35,* 461–470.

# Index